# Fiona's Fight

Fiona Fifield *with* Alisha Jordan

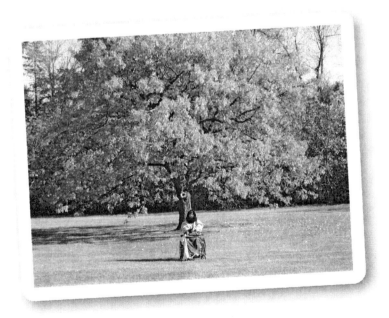

Fiona's Fight
Copyright 2015 by Fiona Fifield

Tellwell Talent
www.tellwell.ca

ISBN: 978-0-9940058-4-7

This Book is dedicated to:

*My Parents, Don & Carol*

*Kyle*

*Ralph*

*Anna*

I Believe In Angels

*'Cause I believe in angels*
*With every breath that I breathe*
*I believe in angels, 'cause my angels believe in me*

—performed by George Canyon

# Contents

# Fiona's Fight

# Fiona

I WAS RAISED ON A LITTLE SLICE OF HEAVEN JUST OUTSIDE OF Caroline, Alberta, two miles south of a remote hamlet called Raven. I was born October 26, 1972 in a small hospital in Innisfail, AB. My birth almost resulted in the death of me and/or my mother. My mother had undiagnosed placental previa, and as a result ended up delivering the placenta before me. You can imagine how fatal this complication can be. As you read on you will see that this was just the first of many close encounters I would have with my demise.

My mother and I came home from the hospital to a 10x28 foot trailer perched on a hill that overlooked my Uncle Gustuv's farmstead. I was welcomed with loving and open arms by my sister, Teena, who was six on the cusp of seven at the time, and an audience of close knit family members whom all lived within thirty miles. My family lived at my Uncle Gustuv's until my father found work on my Uncle Hulger's farm outside of Olds. Eventually, my Uncle Gustuv sub-divided his land and gave three acres to my parents. Uncle Gustuv was my mother's godfather and he took great pride in caring for and assisting my mother. My parents bought a double wide trailer and placed it on the land Uncle Gustuv gifted them. This home would become the highlight of my childhood.

My earliest memories of my mother consisted of baking, blanching vegetables to freeze for the winter and playing cards and other games during rainstorms.

Early memories of my father are few because he worked so hard and was often away. When he was around, I remember sleeping on the floor boards of his truck and decorating the Christmas tree together. When he had time there was always general horseplay and rough housing.

My family has never been wealthy by any means but what we lack financially, we make up tenfold with love and support. I wouldn't have it any other way.

My mother has primary progressive multiple sclerosis (MS) which she was diagnosed with in 1998, and my father has been sick since before my birth. His first spinal surgery occurred just two years after they were married and shortly before the birth of my sister in 1965. My sister was diagnosed with relapsing-remitting MS in 1996, but since has progressed to secondary progressive MS. I was diagnosed with remitting relapsing MS in 2005. As you can see, there is extensive evidence of our ill fortune within the gene pool.

Growing up, I was a normal child with a wonderfully strong family on a hobby farm. The farm brought me immense joy while playing and discovering every square foot. We were always very busy, from gardening to tending to the flower beds and animals, the list would stretch with chores day to day. My sister and I picked raspberries and strawberries, assisting with endless weeding and gardening.

When we didn't have to attend school, a typical day would involve rising at the crack of dawn, gathering eggs and feeding the critters which consisted of chickens, ducks, geese, goats, sheep, cows, pigs, cats and dogs. I remember there were some evenings when I would have to collect eggs after the sun had already set. My fear of the dark made the process terrifying and much quicker.

My father would often be in the garage tinkering, my sister and I would be playing outside while my mother was tending to all of our needs and then some. I laugh at this new age obsession with organics and the viewpoint of its exclusive luxury. I feel fortunate that's the only kind of food I was nourished with and the hard work to produce it was all thanks to us living below the poverty line.

My family cut, split and stacked wood every weekend. One weekend when I was 8 or 9, I was up in the box of my father's truck. Bent over, I picked up pieces of wood and tossed them out between my legs. My mother walked to the back of the truck and bent down to grab a piece of that fell. She stood up as I was chucking a piece out and I completely cold cocked her. She went down for the count. I feel bad when I think of it because she could have been seriously injured. She was fine, just slightly tender on the head.

My mother's parents were immigrants from Denmark. They had very little before they came to Canada. Growing up in poverty herself, my mother believed that being wealthier would have made our lives much easier. She wasn't wrong in thinking so. It must have been so frustrating to raise her children with similar financial circumstances. The statements she absentmindedly made would lead me to believe that we weren't as well off as I believed.

My mother made every scrap of food that ever graced our stomachs from scratch and that included the butchering of our meat.

While providing nourishing meals for her family she also took extra care of my father and his impeding ailments. She also took care of her parents, my grandfather and pyromaniac grandmother. The reason why grandma got the label of pyromaniac was not only for her seemingly insatiable obsession with burning everything and anything, but because in her path of destruction were two homes burned to the ground and many close calls to follow. So, in more words or less and quite blatantly, my mother was a very busy lady.

My mom would not say 'shit' if her mouth was full of it, she is very proper. My sister inherited this grace, I, unfortunately did not. My father is a rowdy, bellowing jokester who is always fun and enjoyable to be around. In early years my mother took him from the dangerous lifestyle that can come with those traits and ultimately saved him. I am my father's daughter, as my sister is my mother's, through and through.

My father, despite his challenging health issues, always worked hard to provide us with what we needed. He drove truck, crafted in woodwork and he would take on numerous odd jobs that his health would permit. He's been a workhorse his entire life. Even though time was sparse between my parents, they were always very united and this provided a good, sturdy foundation for our family. I proudly say I inherited my work ethic from them, almost to a fault.

The chores and work that came with the farm taught me the responsibility and value of hard work later in life. In my youth I was more focused on my own personal needs than the value of anything truly important. However, the work from dusk to dawn never really felt too excessive because we were always surrounded by beautiful countryside scenery. Not only was I surrounded by the beauty of nature but also by my family. A half a mile from the farm lived my Uncle Gustuv and just a few miles from him resided my grandpa and granny. I am blessed to have been able to witness true love first hand from my very own parents. I was also fortunate to have everyone and everything I loved surrounding me from birth.

My Uncle Gustuv was also my mother's brother in law. His wife, Mary, was mother's eldest sister who passed away the year I was born. I never had the pleasure of knowing her but Uncle Gustuv was and will forever be one of the kindest hearted men I've ever known.

Uncle Gustuv was a wiry, compassionate, hardworking man, who was always present in my life. He was an older Danish man who lived in a home with no running water, electricity and used a wood stove. He lived quite modestly, but happily. He and my grandparents played a large role in assisting my parents with child care during my father's more trying health difficulties.

I used to love watching Uncle Gustuv shave. I would watch in wonder as he would heat water on his wood stove, then pour it into a tin bowl and move it to his wash table. This is when he would begin his ritual. He would rub his face with soap using a shave brush that had a brown handle and long bristles. After frothing up his face he would use a straight razor. I was always nervous he would cut himself, but he never did. The best part of watching this was that he let me throw out his water. I would wait through this entire process just so I could dump out that tin bowl.

He was a sinewy man and he used to flex out the smallest, yet defined bicep. This reminded me of Popeye and still makes me snicker just thinking about it. I was at his house often and we would play cards by the hour. As it turned out, I had been playing poker for years before I knew the proper name. We played black jack but at the time he called it 21, we played lots of rummy too. I remember we would sit and chat for hours, rocking on a beautiful wooden swing he built. It was one of those swings that had a large bench seat that could hold about four adults or oodles of children. It was surrounded by Spruce trees that towered around you while swinging comfortably.

I spent a lot of time with Uncle Gustuv while my father was sick in the hospital. I would disembark the bus at his lane instead of mine where he would nurture me during those confusing times.

My father and Uncle Gustuv built my sister and I the most marvellous little play house. It had two rooms with doorways four feet high. Inside was a little kitchen table with two chairs that were red and blue, all hand crafted from wood and the table was built right in under the east facing window. They built the tiny home right along a pathway in the tree lining that lead to the pastures. I can see it perfectly as I reminisce and the vision stirs up sentiments of a better, more carefree time. When I would enter through the small doorway the table would be to my left and the doorway to the second room on my right. The second room was the living room which had two windows too. There my sister and I would play for hours, in an imaginary world which consisted of all of our perceptions about how independent living would be, so very simplistic.

It couldn't have been more perfect, having all of that room to gallivant and play on a roaming landscape which also held a home of our own that fit our size.

Uncle Gustuv would travel back to Denmark every few years and upon returning he would always bring me back a pair of wooden shoes. They had leather binding on the top and a strip of rubber on the soles. They were my favorite, and it wasn't hard to tell by the end of the year, when the soles would be worn down to nothing. I went through three pairs as a child, red, blue and yellow, and I still own a pair from my adulthood, which I treasure, even though I can no longer wear them because of issues I have with my feet swelling.

Teena, my sister, being seven years older, naturally took an authoritative and maternal role with me. She looked out for me while we would play until dark; one of my favorite memories with her was playing badminton on the lawn. We were young and blissfully free children, relishing the summer dusk, and that was the epitome of our lives at the time.

When I was eleven, my sister graduated and left home to join the air force. It made me heartsick, sad and alone. I still saw her in the summers but I was always painstakingly aware of her absence.

Now that I've shed some light into my family and all of their loving support, I will tell you a little bit about the troublesome child named Fiona. I am a very strong-willed individual and I have been since the time I could speak. It seemed once I reached my terrible twos I was stuck in that mindset for a much longer period of time. I am fiercely independent and my belligerent attitude and rejection of anything other than my own way leads me to more trouble than I can handle. A major contribution to my attitude, although intentions were much more pure, was the freedom and sheltered life I was given as a child. I was able to do whatever I wanted, whenever I wanted with little consequence to result. My parents never physically disciplined me, however, looking back they probably should have. My mother's love and my parents concern for sheltering us from the stresses of their own lives, they felt bad disciplining us at all. What you absolutely must know is that my parents are the pillars of strength that have supported and guided me throughout my entire life, even to this day.

They sheltered me from the stress of the comprehension of my father's pain and illness. They did so by leaving me with my grandparents or Uncle Gustuv while my father endured surgery after surgery. For the most part they were successful because I have few recollections of his ailments during this time. They protected me from the horrors of suffering and certain elements that I cannot disclose because they are too closely related. If I had been exposed my story would be entirely different and in a much a darker light. I view my parent's overprotection as a blessing and for this, I thank them. Their upbringing taught me to be strong and independent, proud of who I am and what I can accomplish. The morals and values I treasure were instilled by them, making me who I am today, and this is a fact. I wish I could have acknowledged this earlier, but because of my 'terrible-two' attitude I always felt I needed more. I was selfish to the core.

As I grew up I experienced a sadness that would prolong well into my adolescent years. I lived on the borderline of two districts. All of my friends and family attended Caroline school. I ended up having to attend Spruce View School which was populated by seven hundred and fifty rural children whom I had never connected with before. I was completely disconnected from them, by blood and class. While writing this book, I was confronted by the realization of just how disconnected I really was. How the absence of my family amongst my peers truly impacted me. As I said earlier, we lived well below the poverty line; naturally I didn't fit in at all.

I was young so I was unable to understand why we didn't have as much money as the other children. My entire time at the school I only had a few close friends who happened to also be in the same tax bracket.

With the sadness I also realize I was quite lonely too. Despite the many things I had to be grateful for, the major contributing factor to these feelings was from my father being so sick. As horrible as that may seem, that was the truth. Even with all of the love and attention I received, I only yearned for more. While my mother tended to the needs of my father and my aging grandparents I felt left out. I didn't understand that other people might need more attention, I didn't want to understand. It wasn't that I was unhappy; I was just lonely because I always suffered an insatiable need for individual, undivided attention. With my family, this was not logically possible. Later on during recovery I would recognize this as an addictive behaviour.

My addictive behavior began when I was just five years old. My Granny had a little sealed jar that she kept cigarettes in for when company came over. I took my first cigarette from this jar. I went out to the muskeg and sat on turtle. Turtle was a hump of sod shaped just like; yes you guessed it – a turtle. Turtle was large enough to fit two, possibly three of us. Sitting on top of turtle is where my neighbour Drew and I were busted by my sister smoking the stolen cigarette from Granny's jar. I have no recollection of the result but it makes me aware that my rebellious nature started at a very young age.

Cigarettes would become my nemesis for many years after that first one. When I started to get older I would sneak cigarettes from my father and ride my bike down to a huge culvert that was under the highway and smoke them there.

My first drinking experience was when I was 12 at my cousin's wedding out of town. My parents rarely stayed anywhere very late and when they were leaving I begged to stay longer. They had a camper attached to the bed of a truck that we were staying in nearby so they allowed me. Once they left, a few of my relatives snuck me drinks, I snuck a few on my own too. It didn't take long for me to become tipsy. I don't remember very much of the rest of the evening. My grandma eventually sent me to bed, so I climbed into the camper and passed out. I got up in the middle of the night and must have forgotten where I was. When I exited the camper I walked right off the end of the tailgate and I tumbled down a steep hill. It would have been quite a sight to see.

My next experience with alcohol was immensely worse and happened when I was 14 years old. I was supposed to be figure skating in Caroline, Alberta. The ice thawed and the rink was useless. A girl

I knew from school offered to take me drinking; she had a bottle of whisky behind her seat in her truck. I remember feeling both elated and apprehensive to have that first drink. Curiosity overtook me and I took a swig.

That drink was the beginning of a very volatile relationship alcohol and I would share.

I have no memories of what the day's activities consisted of but, one thing I do remember is by the evening we had picked up a guy I had never met before named Shawn. The three of us drank a twenty six ounce bottle of rye and after the bottle was finished we headed to Shawn's house where he said he had more booze. Upon arriving at his home I was so intoxicated I needed assistance getting inside the house. When I say assistance I mean Shawn had to carry me. I'm unsure of how much time was actually spent at his house but what I do know is that eventually he carried me back out and we were out and about again. My inability to walk must have hindered their fun because it wasn't long before they grew tired of babysitting and tossed me into a snow drift near the arena. The only reason I can tell you this story is because a friend of mine named Hali, and her mother Dolly, were the ones who found me lying on that cold snow drift. If it were not for them I might have frozen to death overnight.

Both Dolly and Hali pulled me out of the snow drift and took me home, dragging me up the stairs to my front door. My father answered the door and the booze could not measure up to the amount of crap I was facing.

"You're drunk!" He said scornfully.

"No Papa! I just have the flu" I lied terribly.

My mother and father put me to bed at first, but not long after they took me to the hospital. They were concerned by the severity of my inebriation. They feared I'd been hurt and/or violated from the blood that was all over my pants. Conveniently, my monthly cycle decided it would be a good time to start that evening. I was so drunk that I didn't even notice. The result of that night was vomiting all over myself while losing my ability to control my bladder and bowels throughout an eighteen hour sleep.

Not long after this episode my father's health worsened. He suffered a grand mal seizure and the straw that broke the proverbial camel's back was that he started having transient ischemic attacks (TIA) which can also be described as 'mini strokes'.

My father's added ailments resulted in us having to leave the solace of the farm, moving thirty miles away to Innisfail to be closer to the hospital. It may not seem very far but at fifteen it felt incredibly overwhelming. I felt as if I had lost everyone I had ever known and loved. These prominent feelings combined with the hormones from being an adolescent with naturally rebellious reserves was a cocktail for disaster.

For the first fifteen years of my life I lived in a safe and stable place surrounded by people who loved and protected me. Now, living in larger town, my mother and father is all I had left, my sister had long been gone.

It was 1989, I was sixteen and I looked like a blonde pinup bombshell. I had cute petite features and an hourglass figure, not surprisingly I ended up hanging out with a bad crowd. I tried hard to fit in, to be liked and wanted, trying to quench my insatiable thirst for attention. Even though Innisfail is not a very large town, it is still vastly different from the farm I grew up on.

Once again, I was in a school longing for acceptance, and the crowd I found were all too happy to corrupt the new naive country girl.

I ended up hanging around with an older man whose family I knew from Caroline. I didn't know him well and sometimes wish I hadn't known him at all. Although he has no blame, it was his house that I endured one of the most horrific experiences of my life.

He had planned a party at his house and hadn't made it back in time to greet his guests because he was with his children. I was alone at the house, hanging out, when everyone started showing up. Nervously trying to calm my nerves, I began drinking. Predictably, being sixteen and apathetic to my own boundaries, I drank way too much.

The memories I have are few but the few I still carry with me I wish I had forgotten.

I remember a football jock named Brett throwing me over his shoulder like a sack of potatoes. I was too intoxicated to think past the moment. I watched the squares of the linoleum floor tick by as he carried me to a bedroom. He threw me onto the bed, and although distorted, I can still feel the pain. I still remember the blood and tears. I can still see the face of the man who took my virtue with force while I was helplessly inebriated.

Following the party, rumors arose that I had had sex while on my cycle. I was being humiliated by the very evidence of my virginity torn from me and left on the sheets. I was made fun of regularly and because of the shame I held for what had happened, I ended up skipping class until finally dismissed from school completely.

Sad, hurt and alone, I told no one, afraid of what pain it might inflict on my parents and what would happen if anyone did find out. I didn't want my father to end up in jail.

My grandfather died shortly after I was kicked out of school in March 1990. My grandmother Larsen was sent to a long term care facility in Didsbury, and my parents to moved there to be closer to her. We couldn't stand the idea that she was all alone. Within a couple of weeks we moved to Didsbury. Shortly after moving and only one month after my grandfather's passing, poor grandma Larsen passed too.

As quickly as I lost my dignity, I lost control of my life. I began drinking heavily and shaming myself beyond anything I could have even imagined possible. I was devastated by the loss of my grandparents and isolated from my peers for being a 'tramp'. Ironically, I ended up becoming just that.

My parents had to watch their daughter throw her life away while completely perplexed as to why. They were grieving as well and they made numerous attempts to help me through counselling and various other resources. I fought them tooth and nail, I couldn't be helped. I refused to divulge my secret and eventually my parents kicked me out. It wasn't for very long though, they loved me too much to follow that plan through.

By May my parents sent me to sign up for the Canadian Reserves in Calgary when I was seventeen. It seemed logical that the disciplinary lifestyle I would learn in the military would help their girl. The intention was good, however, it turns out the Reserves is not a very good place to send an alcoholic. My drinking became even more out of control surrounded by numerous men to shame myself with.

I was desecrated a few more times when I would actually say no.

Surprisingly, I met a few who genuinely loved me, but not feeling worthy of love and therefore unable to love myself; I was incapable of receiving it. Anyone who tried to love me I would merely push away. I was a nice girl who relied on alcohol to save me from having to deal with my own self; it was my best friend, my lover, my all.

I have no recollection under what circumstances I left the reserves. As brutally honest as I can be, my alcoholism had progressed to such a state. Perhaps I should be grateful that I would drink to the point of blacking out completely half past the point of effing oblivion. I don't exaggerate when I describe this either. My alcoholism may have sheltered me from my pain, but it lead me to committing horrific acts, becoming more reprehensible by the day. It put me in situations where I would be violated until I was stripped completely of my dignity, my morals and my very soul. I was an empty shell of a young woman who had lost all self-respect.

I went back to Didsbury to live with my parents again. I reconnected with a girl named Mary whom I met shortly after the first time I was raped. She was a good soul, caught up in the same spiral of intemperance that I was in. It was ironic because she used to escape her broken home to come to my home for solace, and when I wanted to escape my mundanely stable home, I would party at her house. A few years later she would fall in love with Brett, the man who first raped me.

One evening, I was drinking at the Highwayman Motor Inn in Innisfail with friends. I frequented many bars between Red Deer and Calgary, if there was booze, I was there. Oftentimes I would end up in different towns than I had started in.

I had a headache and I asked around for a Tylenol, Gary, a guy I went to school with gave me a little white pill. I don't know what that pill was, but it sure as hell wasn't Tylenol. As soon as that pill kicked in I have no recollection of the rest of the evening.

I woke the next morning in a hotel room, naked on the floor, curled up in the fetal position around the legs of a table. When I finally stood up I saw Brett asleep on the bed. I immediately felt sick to my stomach. I was perplexed how this could possibly happen again. How did I black out and end up being violated again by the man who drove me to my alcoholism in the first place?

I searched for my clothes, finding them in a soaking wet heap on the floor. I put them on anyway and left as quickly as I could. I got in my car and drove straight home. I had no idea that Mary was with Brett at this point. Someone at the bar told Mary about Brett and I leaving together, she never spoke to me again.

I don't blame her for not talking to me and I wish I had had the strength to tell her what was really going on with me. Wherever she is, and if by some chance she ever reads this, I hope that she knows how much I truly care and love her, even to this day. She is a wonderful person that was just another casualty in my downward spiral.

After losing my best friend I did the only thing I knew how to do, drink. I drank copiously and sunk deeper into the abyss of the catastrophe that was my life. I continued to hurt the few people who still stuck around and exceed that hurt more and more.

My dad turned 50 on the 8th of August 1991. I took my folks out to supper for his birthday. We all went to nice restaurant in Olds. I bought a bottle of wine to have with supper. It was a nice dinner with lots of laughs like always. I'm sure that my laughter was a mask and probably blatantly so because it was more belligerent than everyone else's. I was putting on a show to make my father happy. At this point I was getting near the end of my drinking even if I wasn't aware of it at the time.

Moving forward to after the dinner, I got blackout drunk until two days later. Another countless time I woke in a bed not my own, with a man I did not know. I was supposed to be babysitting my Cousin Julie's daughter at 7 that morning. Julie and I worked in the same hotel, she worked the morning shift and I worked the afternoon. While she was at work I would babysit Kari, her baby girl, or at least I was supposed to.

Sadly, on this morning I didn't show. I just laid there knowing that this time I had screwed up beyond forgiveness.

On top of not showing up for my cousin, I remembered I had done something bad the night before. I bumped a car in the parking lot of the bar I was at while trying to leave. I know today, looking back, it really was just a bump. I was too drunk to be driving.

I had a standard car and I was so intoxicated my brain could not coordinate with my feet. I feathered the clutch and fuel pedals at the same time and my car rolled back, bumping into a parked car. I count my blessings it wasn't a person.

Living in a small town it was likely that my dad would have already known of the bump. He always managed to know where I was when I was somewhere I shouldn't be. Always.

He would bang on doors and drag me out of men's houses. Funny, I don't think he knows about the little bump to this day.

I had embellished my own disgraceful actions so much that it terrified me. I don't like to brag but, I pride myself on my driving skills and something as foolish as rolling into a parked car greatly bruised my ego. Nobody knew I bumped the car, but I didn't know that for sure and I thought if anyone did see me, I was done for.

My father would kill me because I had embarrassed and ashamed both my parents enough with my behaviour. This drunk was the final straw and they were done with me. I was done with me.

I crawled out of bed sometime mid-morning. For the first time in my life I had nowhere to go. I wasn't able to go home, I was too embarrassed. I couldn't face my parents or my family now that my alcoholism was completely in the light.

By this point in my drinking career I had no friends left because I had either used them or slept with their boyfriends. Included was a long list of other terrible transgressions. The night I bumped my car was the night I had drank my last drink.

After leaving the strangers house I crawled into my car, sat there and cried. I tried to figure out where I could go to escape the repercussions of my actions. When I could not think of anyone or anywhere that would accept me I realized that my life was not worth living. I was filled with self-pity. I believed the world would be better off without me. Being an alcoholic, I am self-involved by character, but only once have I ever been that selfish.

I drove around the little town of Sundre until I hatched a plan. I was going to drive down a back road and wrap my car around a power pole. I know, stupid plan. It was all I could come up with on short notice. It seemed like it would do the job.

It's funny how things come to light.

While I was writing this someone asked me "why such a violent way to kill yourself?" She stated, "Women normally find much more gentle ways to go out." I hadn't ever thought of it until asked. The truth is, it really was on short notice and I had no more dignity left to spare myself an easy exit out of this world.

I headed north out of town and prayed for God to give me the strength to end my life. I needed to give the people that loved me peace and, at this point, I truly believed if I were gone they would have just that. I sobbed all the way to the pole I planned on ramming into. Never in my life have I felt such deep and utter despair. My last memory was aiming for the pole at the end of the road which also happened to be across a highway, I put my foot on the gas pedal and pressed it to the floor.

The next conscious moment I was heading east on the Bowden highway, God had other plans for me. Just like the song, God had taken the wheel. I turned north and drove to the last place I felt truly happy, where I grew up. I drove by our old acreage knowing it was someone else's little piece of heaven now, and then I cried. I continued to drive. It came to mind that my mom had a friend named Gwen in Innisfail that didn't drink. I still to this day have no idea how I knew that, I just did. I drove to her house and knocked on the door.

When she answered I'm sure I must have looked and smelled like hell. She let me in anyway. I sat on her sofa and wept. Oh my Lord, I cried like never before or since. It was a guttural cry of anguishing loss. I was now painfully aware I had lost everyone and everything including myself.

Gwen insisted I call my folks, even if it was for no other reason than to let them know I was safe. I refused for quite a while, I knew by now they would have learned of my bump.

Gwen took the choice out of my hands and she called. My mom answered and after Gwen interceded in the turmoil she handed me the phone. I could hear my dad yelling in the background; it is amazing how much anger can be produced by fear. They were terrified for their little girl and had been for some time. At 18, I had caused an awful lot of pain and heartache in the last three years.

Mom and I talked for a while, my parents decided to pick me up, my dad would not let me drive my car. The next hour was the longest in my life, waiting for their arrival, the fear of facing my father's wrath and disappointment. There were plenty of both to go around. My dad wouldn't even talk to me let alone look at me he was so angry.

It took him a few days before he could speak to me again. I hadn't had a drink and by that point I was ill from the withdrawals. I asked my parents to keep my return to town a secret because I was so ashamed, especially after my last drinking venture. I was at my rock bottom with a broken soul hiding behind the mask of a drunk degenerate.

My parents put me into one of the rooms in the back row of the motel they were managing in Sundre. I laid in that room for several days detoxing on my own. My mom would bring me food in hopes that I would eat but I couldn't. I tried, but anything that went down would come right back up with sour bile. It was like this for a couple days.

One day my Mom came in and asked me, "Can Julie and a friend of hers come and talk with you?"

Julie had been investigating my welfare and finally I allowed her to visit with a woman who I now refer to as an angel. She's an angel because Julie has no recollection of whom she was or how she found her and I haven't been able to track her down since.

When Julie and the angel came in my room I was lying in bed. They brought a beautiful bouquet of flowers and laid them by my head. I immediately began to cry, I felt so lost, scared, alone and confused. I felt undeserving of their love and support. The angel told me her story of recovery while I wept. It was the first time I registered that I wasn't alone in my struggle. This woman knew exactly what I was feeling and it lifted a weight. It has been 23 years since that day and neither Julie nor I can remember the name of that angel of a lady. I think she was from Calgary but I honestly have no idea how or where Julie found her, all I know is that my life has never been the same since.

Everything following that visit all happened very fast. I think my unknown angel set up my quick admittance into the Detox Centre. I was dropped off there the very next day. My mom had driven me and the fear and apprehension of getting sober was all consuming. I was terrified to get out of the car. I knew the moment I walked into that building I would never be the same person again. I sobbed and hugged my mother tightly you would have thought I was walking a plank.

I finally found the courage to release my mom. She had been my rock all of my life, I leaned on her for so long. Now, we were both tired and ready for things to change. I needed to grow up and try to move forward with my life. I got out of the car and walked to the entrance. There was a button to push to be let in; I knew it would be much harder to get out. Once I pushed the button I looked back at my mom and the tears flowed from both of us.

An intake worker came and opened the door. I walked through the door with suitcase in hand. The worker sat me down and asked me a raft of questions. It was all a daze. They went through my suitcase and took my perfume, my hairspray and anything with alcohol in it. I was growing irritated and acting snotty at this point of the process.

I was stunned and I said "why are you taking my stuff away? That is mine, you have no right."

This was my first lesson; it had to be locked away because they thought I or someone else may drink it. I was appalled at the idea of such a thing.

She said, "People do it all the time."

"That's nuts it could kill you!" I said

She nodded, "This is the difference between getting sober at eighteen and doing it later."

I was learning things about alcoholism that I couldn't fathom. I thought it was absolutely ludicrous that anyone might consume hairspray or perfume and I should have those privileges because I wasn't that desperate. I went into rehab thinking I was somebody special, thinking I was a tough chick from Caroline. I quickly found out that my drinking was nothing in comparison to some of the people I would meet there. There was nothing special about me at all.

They performed a routine health examination, checked my blood pressure and pulse. Then they put me into the rubber room. (That is what they call it!) It is a room with beds across the hall from the intake office. It is where you endure the worst of the physical detox. They needed to be able to keep a close eye on me while I suffered. I thought the time I spent in that motel room would have been enough physical detoxing for me, but they obviously didn't think so. It was in the rubber room when I figured out I would never drink again.

I witnessed people doing things that I still find hard to believe. They were in a state of utter delusional suffering and it terrified me. Some saw spiders on the walls, covering them. I sincerely thought that they would die from the way they were wailing. It gave me an idea of where I could have ended up. Thankfully, I was only in that rubber room for a couple of days.

I was transferred from the rubber room to a main building for another week. I took part in group meetings and was treated like a hyperactive child; there were caffeine restrictions at certain times of the day. There was a pool table and TV with workbooks to fill out. The following week was when I went to my first in-house meeting for a twelve step program. It was this program where I realized how bad my drinking had actually affected me.

I spent nine very informative and clarifying days in detox.

My mother picked me up, I was nervous that if I went home between detox and treatment that I would be sure to drink again. I wasn't very confident in my abilities to stay sober.

After arriving back in Didsbury, I went to my very first meeting. I was picked up by an older gentleman by the name of Harold. Harold showed up at my parent's door with my first Big Book, I still have it today. This is the book that would forever change my life and my perspective.

My mom took me on a mini vacation to keep me busy until I could get into a 28 day treatment program.

My life was altered for the better when I acknowledged I was slowly killing myself by drinking my young self to death. I have no real reason for becoming an alcoholic other than the fact that it was in my genetic makeup. My immediate family had no trace of the disease, but there certainly was some in earlier generations. It's very rare that you find alcoholics who don't already have one or two in the woodshed.

I often look back at this time, and every day since I have been eternally grateful for having been saved by my sobriety. Without the start of my relationship with my higher power I would never have been able to handle what my life was soon to become. I would not have been prepared for how much change and growth would be required to deal with the major health challenges I would be facing.

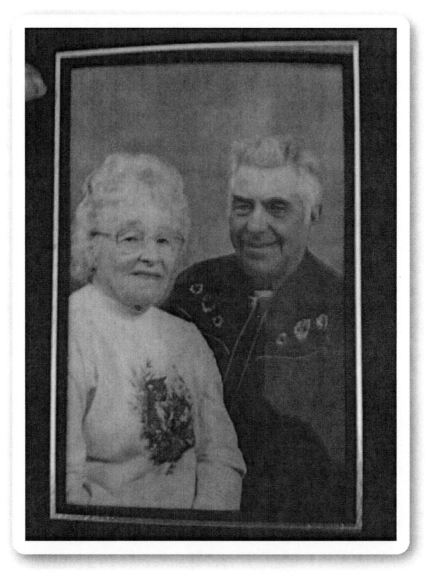

*Grandma and Grandpa Jones, (my dad's parents)*

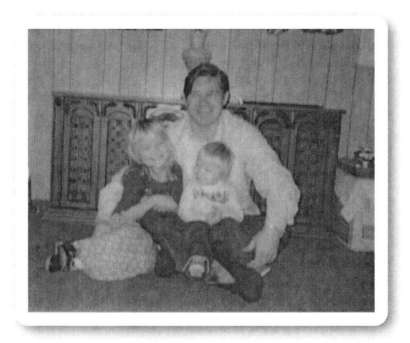

*Dad, Teena and I*

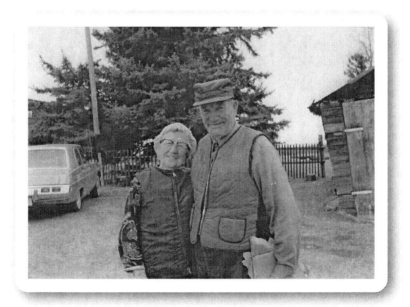

*Grandma and Grandpa Larsen*

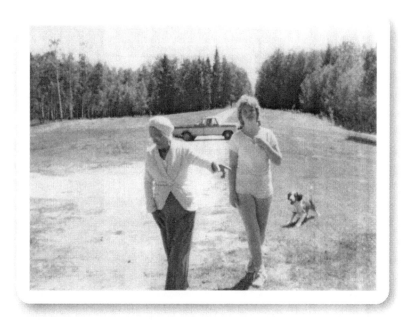

*Grandma Larsen and I*

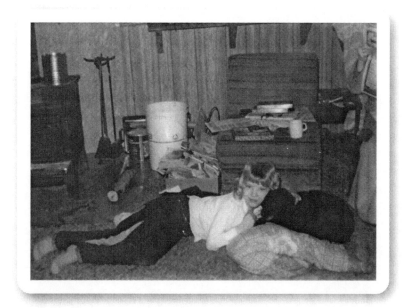

*Me and my dog Angie*

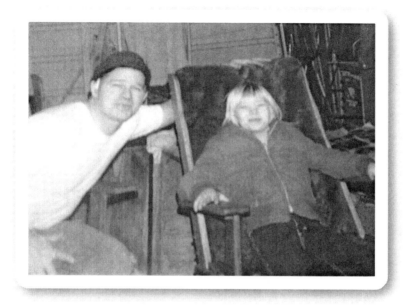

*Me and my father. I'm sitting in the chair he built*

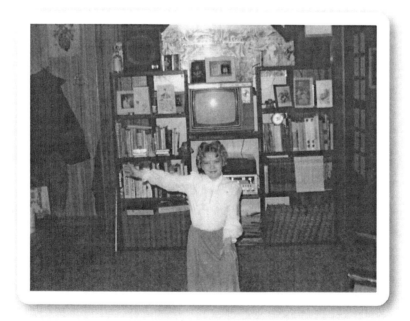

*Me in my figure skating outfit, eat your heart out*

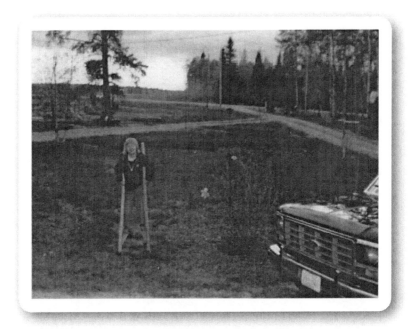

*Me standing on stilts in the yard*

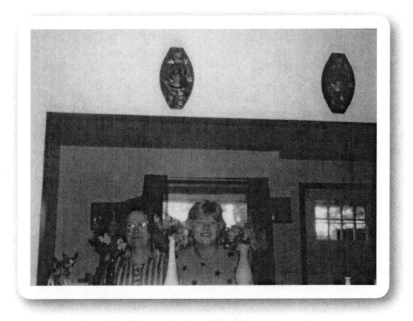

*Mom and I behind our fresh picked sweet peas*

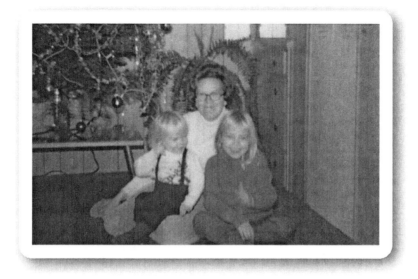

*Mom, me and Teena*

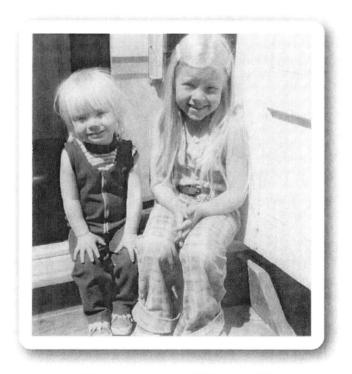

*My favorite picture of Teena and I*

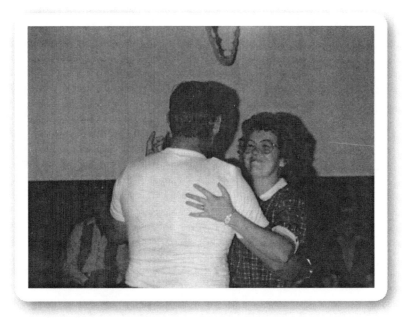

*My mother and father dancing, while they still could*

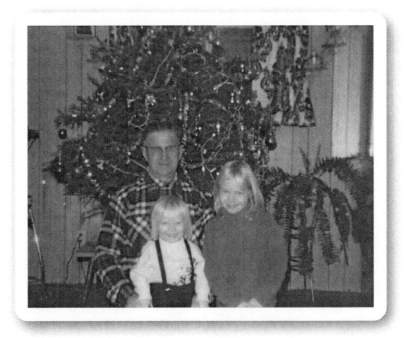

*Uncle Gutuv, me and Teena*

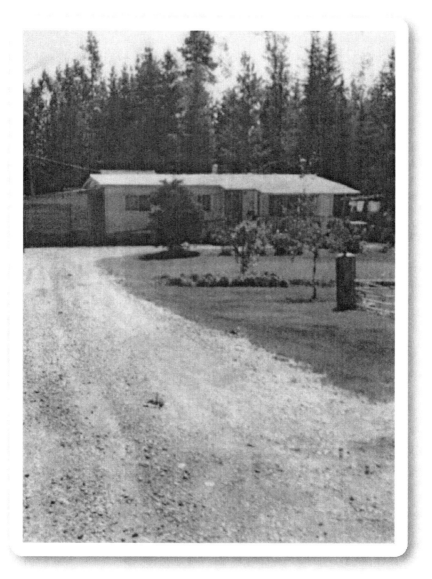

*The hobby farm I grew up on*

# The Twelve Steps and the Journey in Between

MY EARLY TIME IN SOBRIETY WAS NOT EASY ON ME, AT LEAST I believed so. I was still young and I received a lot of attention attending meetings, but my desire for attention was insatiable. I still had a lot of growing up to do. Once I sobered up there were a multitude of issues that I found myself caught up in. I was back home, living with my parents in Didsbury, going to meetings and doing my best to stay out of trouble. At the meetings I met a man named Ralph and a woman named Linda. They quickly became dear and close friends, members of my family, who played a massive role in my support to stay sober. Linda Lou is a great companion and we kept each other sober, but still managed to get into trouble. Ralph was crazy, I loved him so.

Ralph, Linda and I would go to meetings in Olds on Mondays

and Tuesdays, Wednesdays in Sundre, Thursdays we would take off and Friday to Sunday we would go to Didsbury or Calgary to attend sober dances. We attended roughly eight meetings during the week and five on weekends. In one year we went to well over four hundred meetings.

My favorite memory of Ralph was walking with him in the shallow Little Red Deer River. We would remove our shoes and socks, roll up our pants and saunter down the river. It was calming and peaceful and we would talk all the while.

I ended up having a brief relationship with a young man by the name of Al. It was a loveless relationship and we had hooked up in my drinking days, his house was one of the houses my dad dragged me out of. We lived together but ended up severing the relationship because of the lack of love. I can't say I ever felt truly connected to any man by this point and certainly didn't love any.

I moved to a farm just outside Cremona to take a nanny job. I worked from 7am to 5pm and then Ralph and I would go to meetings. I loved meetings because they were reminders that I wasn't the only troubled soul. It made me feel good to be around people who understood where I was coming from. I wasn't being judged or ridiculed, I was accepted. This is how I always felt when I was with Ralph. He tolerated everything about me and loved me even more for my flaws. Without him I would not be sober today. I was wild and belligerent with no filter and the mouth of a trucker long before I became one.

Ralph was hands down, my very best friend, through thick and thin. We lived on peanuts, bags and bags of salted peanuts.

I was a lot like a chameleon in the aspect that I blended and fit in with all sorts of people and crowds. In the meetings, there was Linda Lou and the bikers, the cowboys who were people after my own heart, the yuppies whom I really wanted to be like and the regular Joe blows with families and jobs. I hung out with all of them whenever they were around and they all accepted me as the wild card.

One evening Ralph and I attended a sober dance and every single clique was there, which really didn't happen often.

Ralph turned to me and said, "Fiona, I have a question for you," I looked to him, "Can you tell me who you're going to be tonight?"

"What the fuck do you mean?" I was taken aback.

"Well, all the groups are here. You're this way with these people and that way with those people, who are you going to be with them all here?"

Mildly offended and flabbergasted, I realized he was right. This was the first day I really started looking in the mirror. I had been hanging out with Ralph from '91-'95, for four years by this point, and I didn't see how much I was still flailing out of control. Sober but still lost and unsure of whom Fiona really was as a person. I am grateful that Ralph loved me anyway, unconditionally.

I was in treatment with a young woman named Margaret and we hit it off instantly. We were lunatics, two nuts in a nutshell. Margaret, whom I called Maggie May, and I were twins in looks and personality. We were the shit disturbers at the meetings, constantly getting into trouble.

For a few years we weren't as close because I lived far away and we were at different crossroads in our lives.

We ended up reconnecting in '93 and decided to get a place together in Calgary. I had fallen in 'love' with a man named Bill who lived in Calgary and I was moving to the big city to be near him. Maggie and I got an apartment in North Mount near Confederation Park and continued to go to meetings together. As quickly as I moved to Calgary to be with Bill, he dumped me even quicker. We were never really together, I pined for him but he led me on until he had completely used me up. Keep in mind; though I was sober, I still had the same habits of self-seeking as when I drank. It was imprinted inside me from before I can remember and not that easy for me to recognize or correct.

Early in sobriety I found myself becoming sickly. I was waitressing and going to school to be a class 1 truck driver. I came home from work one evening and soaked my feet. I noticed that two of my toes had turned black.

I went straight to the doctor the next day and where I was diagnosed with [1]Buerger's disease. This disease is rare and effects the arteries and veins in arms and legs, blood vessels become inflamed, swell and can become blocked with blood clots. This eventually damages or destroys skin tissues and can lead to infection and gangrene. I was booked for an amputation of the affected toes. I was terrified when I got the news. I followed every direction that was given, like eating lots of cayenne. My parents bought me a pair of mukluks from Alaska; a woman from the meetings knitted me a blanket to keep my feet warm. I did not, however, quit smoking which is the most crucial necessity for Buerger's disease.

I met a trio of older gentlemen at different meetings. One resembled Santa Claus and all of them were very humorous.

They took me to a spiritual event with some friends. It was strange because it was an older warehouse district of the city. I felt nervous and scared when we walked in and the minister was speaking of someone with bad feet. Paranoid, I believed my friends had told them about me prior to us getting there, they hadn't. I sat and listened to the minister talk. My friends took me up to the front of the room where a bunch of people laid their hands on me and prayed. I stood there astonished I was even there. It felt surreal and I thought they were all nuts.

---

[1]    Information Source: http://www.mayoclinic.org/diseases-conditions/buergers-disease/basics/definition/con-20029501

My opinion of those people changed overnight because when I went to see my specialist next, my toes were no longer black. Magically, my feet were good and my toes no longer needed to be amputated.

As you read on you will see that this is the first of many miracles to come.

I was still broken within my heart, soul and spirit. I met a man named Junior while waitressing at a truck stop. He would come in and spend more time than he should in my section. We became flirtatious acquaintances and one evening after he had left, I found his information written on a napkin underneath the tip he left me. I was taken aback by this, and not wanting to seem desperate, I waited a few days before calling him. He was in the process of getting a divorce and father to two beautiful boys that I absolutely adored. He was my first love, that kind of infatuation that's intoxicating and makes your very soul ache.

Maggie and Ralph would join us for cards games and on my days off I would sit in the passenger seat during his runs. I was with him any and every chance I could. It was the most stable relationship I had ever had. It was real and normal, I cannot emphasize that enough. He treated me like gold and I was on top of the world.

Seven months into our relationship his ex-wife grew jealous of my relationship with the boys and she told him that if he didn't end it between us he would never see his kids again. He was too good of a man to consider me over his children; this only made me love him more. I was left utterly heartbroken.

Three months later I met a man named Ruby at a meeting that Ralph and I attended together often. It was a popular meeting for low-bottom drunks and the setting was usually rather dejected. I stood out being the outgoing, funny and friendly bubbly blonde, which is how I liked it. I did not fit in with this crowd; some accepted me but most resented my nature.

Ruby and I were complete opposites, I was little and fair skinned while he was big, burly and copper. I liked to work the coffee counter at the meetings as a chance to meet everyone and that's how Ruby and I met.

I was still quite heartbroken over Junior and Ruby was there to coddle me, distract me from my sorrow. He asked me to a dance some months later and, for a 6'2" brawny man, he was quite light on his feet. My love for dancing was an easy ticket to my heart. We dated on and off, sharing a volatile relationship for almost six years.

Ruby and I loved each other in a toxic way. Our first year together was blissfully perfect. I moved in with him within a few months after we started dating. It was a small crumby shoebox of an apartment in a scummy part of town. I was so enamored, I left my beautiful apartment I shared with Maggie and moved onto hooker stroll. Shortly after, Ruby and I were engaged but, it was cancelled after the first year when his twelve year old son, Bone, came to live with us.

Bone was a troublemaker. When Bone moved in I realized that

Ruby liked to talk the talk but could hardly walk the walk. His son was out of control. Bone stole my cigarettes and would take off on me while we were at the mall. It broke my heart and still breaks my heart that he was so damaged. Beneath the surface of this little hellion was a heart of gold with absolutely no idea how to display it.

Ruby and I had completely different perspectives to begin with and that alone made us clash constantly. He had no idea how to treat a woman like me, and I think I was the first that tried to demand his respect. We were constantly battling and testing each other's wills to prove one another's love. It was absolute madness. Adding Bone to the equation is where things went completely off track. Bone would play us off of each other while we were already doing that in the first place. I had witnessed first-hand, true and undying love from my parents and neither of these boys had a clue. I had come close with Junior. I guess I had expectations that somehow Ruby would wake up one morning and understand everything I wanted for our relationship. Everything I had had with Junior.

It didn't happen and I realize now that I didn't fall in love with Ruby, I fell in love with his potential. I remember calling my sister close to the end of our madness and she said that if I picked up a drink she would beat me to death with the bottle.

I was five years sober and still hadn't completed step four of the twelve steps. For everyone who is unaware of what step four is: it is facing an honest self-reflection. I had an easy enough time with step one, which is admitting that I have an allergy of the body and an obsession of the mind to alcohol. I really struggled with step two which is having trust that a power greater than myself can restore my sanity. I had a hard time with this because I couldn't understand why God would seemingly bestow such hardships upon me and my family. I could only ask why? I would think about it over and over and I just couldn't grasp it. Step three was making a decision to turn my will and life over to the care of God as I understood him.

I believed I had completed these steps but it wasn't until I completed step four that I realized I hadn't really completed two or three.

Sitting down in front of the mirror and picking yourself apart is a challenge for the best of us. Boy, was it hell for me. I decided to make a serious attempt in confronting my inner demons. What I found was an abundance of selfish and sometimes immoral tendencies, strong resentments with myself and God, an illogical fear of judgment and a plethora of inappropriate sexual conduct.

My selfish tendencies stretched as far back as when I was a young child. My father was facing a lot of challenges with his health and I would pray to God, asking him to take my father to heaven and release him from his pain. I didn't see how selfish this request was and the truth is, deep down I wanted him to take my father so I wouldn't have to hurt anymore.

I heard my mother cry, likely because she was unable to help him and felt helpless. This too made me sad and I didn't want to be sad.

This realization made me feel more resentful towards myself, which was already another problem I had. I held a lot of animosity towards myself for being the way I was, and I blamed God for not making it easier, not just for me but everyone around me.

My fear of judgment was painstakingly blatant in all of my actions. I was constantly pining for attention and ironically, it rooted back to my selfish tendencies.

It was very painful reflecting on my past sexual behaviours.

I was shocked at the complete lack of respect I had for myself. I also understood why and when I first started to hate myself. The first time I was violated had been the root of all the promiscuity, all the booze and degradation. I had told so many lies and kept so many secrets. I was deeply ashamed while confronting these demons.

I cried for hours while facing these truths and in a way it was purifying. I finally gained knowledge of awareness. I had perspective on my life and now I could finally attempt to control it.

With the acknowledgment of step four I was equipped to become the person I am today. It took much longer than just acknowledgment to practice it in my daily life and I mean a lot of practice. But I was aware that this would be the key to my success.

Step five consisted of revealing my secrets to another and my higher power. The purpose of revealing my secrets would relieve me of the burden that I had carried lonesome for so long. That's exactly what it did, immediately after sharing my burdens; it released me from my shame. I was able to forgive myself and look towards the future. For the first time in my life I was able to look at myself in the mirror, really look at myself. And For the very first time in what felt like an eternity, I could look myself in the eye without seeing the looming shame that overshadowed my existence.

Step six concerns the removal of defects of character. My first interpretation was that I was indeed defective. Once again, another misconception produced by my low self-worth. I wasn't picking out the bad traits; I was just combining them as a whole and I couldn't comprehend how to separate the bad habits from myself as a person. I realized that much of the decisions I had made in my life were made from fear. I felt it was absolutely essential to protect myself; self-preservation was always my motivator, although the motivation didn't inspire many good habits.

Confronting my fear forced me to face the hard truth that I yearned to be sicker than I really was. I was constantly judged on not being a 'true' alcoholic because my circumstances weren't as nefarious as they should have been. I told myself that I was a liar, a thief, a con, a cheat and these were the prerequisites to being a 'true' alcoholic. Don't get me wrong, I was many of those things but I didn't end up in a recovery program as a direct result from any of those actions. I joined the twelve step program so my parents would like me, not because it was court ordered, but because I needed to gain back respect.

I stayed long enough to learn that, even with mild alcoholism I was worth being there, despite the criticisms.

Today I look at the defects in my character simply as the seven deadly sins. They all equate to one thing: selfishness. From my perspective, many of the people around the recovery groups want to be sicker, different – set apart from everyone else. While we are taught that the root of our disease is, low and behold, selfishness. We are brought together as group of individuals who have the same life problem but we all seem to focus on the defining points of how we got there. Like we're in a competition to see who is the most effed up because that would make us more deserving of the recovery. If you are like me, not that dysfunctional, then you are a teeny bopper in the world of alcoholics, nobody special.

So as I reviewed my character flaws I found myself perplexed. I didn't come from a dysfunctional household and I had a lot of support. My alcoholism was a direct result from my own damaging predispositions.

My mother often told me, "Fiona, you have champagne taste on a beer budget."

Boy, was that the truth. I always wanted more than I could afford. It was just my nature. Unlike many of the abused and depraved alcoholics, I was a victim to my own hand, I was literally my own worst enemy and I had nobody else to blame.

Step seven was about learning to be humble and asking the higher power to humbly remove my shortcomings. Ironically to be truly humble, you won't be aware that you are humble. Humble was a word I knew absolutely nothing about. This step was a blessing because I was able to look and find humility in others. Seeing people display acts of kindness for no other reason than to be kind was astonishing. I had never thought to be so selfless. I watched a man walk down a street placing a quarter in every parking meter he walked past. Seeing this left me both ashamed and inspired. I was, for the first time in my life, open to seeing kindness in others. I was able to view the good in the world and it opened me up to believe that there are more good people than bad. This is how it will always be. I had chosen to surround myself with the shady folks from the other side of the fence. The power to be surrounded by good people had been in my hands all along and now I sought them out, feeling worthy of being among them.

I relearned that through all of the heartbreak with Junior and all the mess with Ruby, I am still a decent person. I am worthy of self-love and forgiveness.

I wanted to be a truck driver and Ruby didn't want me to drive truck. He thought I would be unfaithful while on the road. His insecurities were rooted from his own unfaithful inclinations. I left him in 1997 and finished my truck driving course with honors; my first job was hauling gravel.

I could have been hauling manure, it wouldn't have mattered, driving brings me a joy that nothing else can. Something about being on the road, behind the wheel makes me feel free, powerful and alive. It brings out the strength in my character and spirit. I'm a damn good driver and it wasn't hard to tell.

I did have one horrific experience and if it weren't for the people in my recovery program I would have ended my driving career before it started.

I got offered a job placement through the school after I graduated. I shared driving duties with an older man in his sixties and we were headed from Calgary all the way to Dallas, Texas. He was ancient with a big white beard but he seemed nice enough. One night at 3am while I was asleep in the bunk, he was supposed to be driving. I woke up to rough, grubby hands shoved down the front of my pants. Terrified, my heart raced a mile minute while I tried to grasp what was happening.

I shoved him off of me and while in hysterics said something to the effect of, "get off of me! Don't you ever touch me again!"

I scurried out of the truck and ran to a payphone. I did the only thing I knew how to do and that was calling someone in the recovery program for support. They had a kind stranger from the program pick me up immediately and take me to a safe place. I am so thankful for the twelve step call because two strangers, in an entirely different country, came to my rescue and took me for coffee before taking me to their house for a rest. I stayed with them for two days until it was time to go back to Calgary. I was in a predicament too because I had no choice but to get back in the truck with the creep to get home. I certainly couldn't afford any other means of travel. The kind Samaritans dropped me back off with him where I cautiously stayed in the front of the truck the entire trip home. When I wasn't driving I was asleep in the jumper seat with one eye open. He didn't say a word to me about it; the most infuriating part was that he acted as if nothing had happened.

It was the first time in my life I had stuck up for me and my morality. The incident changed my perspective on wanting to drive, it took me a whole year after to face my fear and just do what I truly wanted to do, drive. It was conflicting for me, because of my past behaviour; I had a hard time distinguishing if I had provoked the old pervert or was violated by a bad person. With the help of my recovery program and my slow but steady healing and progress, I was able to acknowledge right and wrong. I pursued what I wanted and I was proud that I had attained my job on my merit, not my ass.

After my year hiatus from the scare with the creep I drove gravel truck for two years. I met a man named Tim in the program in 1998 and we dated for a year before getting engaged in 1999. After we were engaged I took a new job on the highway, long haul running team. A running team is when there are dual drivers so that truck can run non-stop. I ran because I needed to learn the ropes of the highway, and also to get past my fear of Mr. Creep and the road itself. It taught me a lot about myself and the kind of person I wanted to be. I was teamed up with both a male and a female and I learned more lessons from the woman than I ever did from the man. She was the prime example of what I didn't want to be, ever. She liked to use her looks and her assets to get her work done for her. In fact, she focused more on her looks than her job. She didn't have an attitude to learn and grow, but rather to exploit herself and let someone else take on her work for her. It disgusted me, especially because I was so familiar with that kind of behaviour.

I was planning a wedding, which is a generally difficult task, but planning it from 3000 miles away was ridiculous. It was the most stressful occurrence I had ever experienced at that point in my life, promiscuity and alcoholism aside. I've always been a go-getter and Tim was a fence-sitter. I had all this drive and motivation to get our wedding under way and he was happy to let me take over. With my new career on the highway always miles away from home, and now a relationship that was relatively new and moving quickly, I was up to my ears in hectic.

Tim and I were married on June 24, 2000. I had a beautiful enormous ruffled white gown with a six foot train. The whole event was charming, it was my dream wedding. The bridesmaids' dresses were royal purple. My maid of honor was my very dear friend Darlene; my bridesmaids were my sister and another woman I met in the program.

We were married in a church and had our reception in a nice hotel venue. There were around two hundred of our close family friends in attendance and we still didn't invite everyone we wanted to.

The most important detail of my wedding was my father. He has been in a wheelchair since I was a teenager and when he found out that I was to be married, he practiced walking with his prosthesis every day. For months he suffered just so he would be able to walk me down the aisle. It meant, and still means the world to me. This is just a small statement of the kind of man my father is.

As I walked down the aisle, on my father's arm, I knew Tim was not the 'one'. Not an ideal time or place for that realization, but from the moment we were married I knew I was not completely invested. It didn't stop me from trying to ignore those feelings and be a good wife though.

The following winter I was in Southern California and it was pouring rain. I sat in Fontana in my truck waiting for the lumber yard to open. After everyone arrived and I got unloaded I saw an adorable, high wired puppy running around the yard like a lunatic. I fell in love with her from that first moment of seeing her. I played with her and bullshitted with one of the yard guys as I waited for my trailer. I returned to my truck to pull out to close my doors and then I jumped back out to close everything else up. I walked up to my truck after the paperwork was signed and there is this damn puppy, covered in mud, sitting up on my seat staring down at me. The boys from the yard made a decision to send me home with my newfound love. They put some cardboard down and placed the very soon to be named, Mahogany, in my truck. I turned and there were around ten guys standing watching me.

"What the hell is this?" I said with a sheepish grin.

Smiles all around, I learned that she didn't belong to anyone. She was a stray that had appeared one day all beat up. They locked her in the gates at night to keep her safe and shared their lunches to keep her fed. They took her in and she had resided with them ever since. They had no idea how old she was and it didn't matter much to me. I needed to save the underdog, what a cheesy pun.

I called dispatch to let them know I was going to be smuggling home a puppy. I asked if they could get me a straight load of bananas back to Calgary. What this meant was, it's illegal to smuggle unregistered creatures across an international border. By asking for a straight load of bananas from Port Hueneme meant that it was a straight crossover to Canada with only one border to cross. Normally, this wouldn't be such a huge request as we do this every day. But with the bananas came apples and three more crossings. Long story short, I ended up having to cross the international line with this little puppy three times before arriving back in Calgary. I called my husband many times during the process of getting Moh home. We had veterinary appointments to make because she had been hurt very bad in Fontana before being saved by the yard men. My guess is she was intended to be fighting dog. I'm grateful Moh was so cute that the first two border protections gave her treats and waved us through.

This little creature instantly became my best friend.

My fondest memory of Moh was her first experience with snow. We were all the way up in northern Idaho. I was a bit panicky because we were at the last illegal crossing before getting back into Canada. I had to get her home and make her a Canadian dog. I pulled over to grab a coffee and let Moh out for a run. She ran into a huge snow drift and I've never laughed so hard in my life. Never feeling snow before, she leapt and bound at a hundred miles an hour, completely covered in it, jumping in and out, weaving excitedly. Watching genuine innocence and joy was refreshing. I watched her for a good twenty minutes before rounding her up and crossed my fingers as we would be crossing our last border soon.

Moh and I made it safely across the border without a fuss.

Once home in Canada, Tim and I had Moh in to see the vet. We were informed Moh was between 6 and 9 months, a large mixed breed of pitbull, Jack Russell Terrier and Hound. I'm sure you're trying to visualize that mish-mash of breeds, but boy was she cute. You wouldn't know there was hound in her until she started to coo at something she desired. She was a severely abused pup before the boys in the yard stumbled upon her. She had a hernia and two teeth kicked out. It broke my heart to think people could beat such an adorable and innocent creature. She was absolutely terrified of men and that was heart wrenchingly sad for me. When I had her fixed they also performed a surgery to fix the hernia. She became my child and I would not enter any place she wasn't welcome thereafter.

My marriage with Tim, sadly, only lasted a year.

I loved him as a person but I was not in love with him. Being the kind of person I am I could not stay with him knowing I could never reciprocate his love. He deserved better than that. I was devastated because I desperately wanted to be the wife he wanted and deserved. Mentally I didn't know how and physically I couldn't. I had unintentionally portrayed myself to be a person that I believed I was capable of being, but the truth always catches up with us. So I moved out after a year and Ralph and I got an apartment. Things were starting to become clearer to me, I was still not very humble and still making mistakes but at least this time I was aware. This was the result of completing the program mid-grade. Slowly but surely things fall into place, but it takes time, a painful process – at least for this alcoholic.

Step eight was about writing down a list of people I owed amends and step nine was becoming willing to do so. Step nine was the most challenging. I had to face all the people I had wronged and then admit I was wrong. The first people I made amends with were my family which was easy, they loved me unconditionally.

They took me for my word when I said, "I'm so sorry, I don't want to be this person anymore and I will do everything in my power to change." This initial acceptance helped me with the start with the rest of my list.

The most meaningful person I made amends with was Ruby. I

didn't do this until 2013. Perhaps I haven't mentioned it yet, but the twelve steps are an ongoing process, even over twenty years later, I am still practicing these steps today.

Ruby was the one to approach me to make amends. We ended up helping each other.

He sent me a message on Facebook asking if we could have lunch the next time I was in the city. I agreed because I never held any real resentment towards him. I'm not a resentful person; it's never been in my nature other than with myself or God.

A few weeks later I picked him up from his home and we went to a Denny's restaurant. For the first time ever, he bought me lunch. Seeing him all those years later made me feel sad for him because I could see he had been abusing himself. Here I had been making exponential progress in my recovery and he was still stuck exactly where I had left, if not worse.

Being that it had been so long, physically I knew exactly who he was, but his soul had changed. His spirit had withered and you could see he was worn from his long struggle.

During lunch he asked me if I needed anything from him, including apologies for the past experiences we shared. I didn't need anything from him, nothing at all, I was content. I think it eased him to know this too. Seeing that I could absolve him of the regrets and remorseful actions that commenced between us was a weight lifted equally from both of our shoulders. The very knowledge of knowing that there were no hard feelings harboured made it so we could cross each other off our lists for step nine.

The last three steps are referred to as the maintenance steps. The only way to be completely done the twelve steps is to become, miraculously, a perfect human being. Step ten is continuing to take personal inventory and when wrong promptly admit it. This step is still a challenge for me. My pride takes over, which in turn causes me to go back to step four. I am who I am and I still have tendencies. I'm not as conscious with this step as I should be, mainly because I'm human and I have higher expectations for myself. I expect better from myself and I feel awful when I can't measure up to the perfection I believe this step implies. In reality, it is just there to make us conscious we can be better. So I guess it serves its purpose, it's just awfully frustrating for me.

Step eleven is giving faith to a higher power and having faith in the outcomes.

[2]The Peace Prayer of Saint Francis

"O Lord, make me an instrument of Thy Peace!

Where there is hatred, let me sow love.

Where there is injury, pardon.

Where there is discord, harmony.

Where there is doubt, faith.

Where there is despair, hope.

Where there is darkness, light.

Where there is sorrow, joy.

Oh Divine Master, grant that I may not

so much seek to be consoled as to console;

to be understood as to understand;

to be loved as to love;

for it is in giving that we receive;

it is in pardoning that we are pardoned;

and it is in dying that we are born to Eternal Life."

I am not a religious person but I am spiritual. This prayer is the complete embodiment of what I believe to be a perfect person. This prayer reminds me of who I want to be and motivates me to strive for that every day.

---

2      Source: http://www.catholic.org/prayers/prayer.php?p=134

Step twelve is affirmation with our higher power, to be better and to spread this knowledge, giving back for all of what we have received. In my opinion this step is not just to help alcoholics; it is to help everyone in any situation. To be the best person I can be. I practice love and tolerance in all aspects of my life, genuinely without hypocrisy, to the best of my ability.

It took me five years to complete steps one through four, another three years to get to step twelve but step nine is still incomplete. Practicing these steps in all my affairs brought me closer to the enlightenment with the immoral actions that I bestowed and were bestowed upon me.

Nearly a decade after the rape I finally sought help for myself. I confided in counsellors, as well as my sponsor and I even helped other girls with some of the same issues while sponsoring them. I never told my family, I don't think I ever would have if I hadn't started writing this book. I even stopped writing it when I realized that I would either have to lie or reveal my secret. I stopped writing out of fear and shame. If my father had known at the time what had happened to me, he would still be in jail. I was ignorant to many things growing up but I never questioned the limits of my parents love. An insidious act such as what happened to me could make a docile and gentle man like my father a killer.

It was not until the spring of 2013 that I was able to share the rape with my sister. There had been a story on the news out of Ohio of a girl who was going through exactly what I had gone through. She was raped by a young man at school and in the process of charging him. I admired her courage. I had long forgiven my perpetrator since the incident; it was part of the process for my steps. I do not condone keeping quiet but I also won't condone harbouring resentments, I know firsthand how much damage can be self-inflicted when you do. I was aware upon writing these memoirs that my mother and sister would be the first to read it. It didn't feel right to reveal such sensitive information to them through a book that would be viewed by quite possibly millions of strangers. I felt stuck so I phoned my sister. I'm not sure why, we'd had such a tumultuous relationship over the years.

"There's something I have to tell you?" I said feeling very anxious.

"What is it?"

"There's been something on the news, the girl in Ohio who was raped. I can't write the book anymore" I said stumbling over my words, not knowing where to begin.

"What are you talking about?" she was puzzled.

"The same thing happened to me and I haven't told anyone about it" I waited in silence for her reaction.

"Fiona" I could hear the lump in her throat, "Why wouldn't you tell me?"

"I didn't feel you had my back" I admitted, surprised she believed me without hesitation.

"I've always had your back, from day one" she said sincerely.

I was in tears, completely reprieved.

All these years she had probably believed I was just a spoiled rotten brat acting out. Now, finally, after over twenty years she had the full truth and realization that my actions were from extenuating circumstances. If I would have known that this revelation would have brought us closer, I might have told her sooner. The past twenty years might not have been so hard on us both.

I have had many such awakenings throughout my sobriety. I thank my higher power every day for giving me the eye openers that I need when I need them.

My sister and I decided that it was best to tell my mother. I knew I had to be very careful about how I told her because it was very important to me that she not believe that she was at fault in any way.

It was mother's day and my mother and I were going out to buy bedding-out plants from the nursery. We got in our electric wheelchairs and decided to cruise across the street. On our way over I looked at her and something inside me told me that it was time to tell her.

As we were rolling along I pulled up beside her and I said, "Mom, there's something I need to tell you from a long time ago that you won't want to hear, but it will explain a lot."

She said, "Go ahead and tell me what you need to tell me"

I got teary and I said, "I just need you to know you are not at fault. Somebody hurt me a long time ago and this is what happened."

She listened intently while I revealed the dark secret which had spun my life out of control. Just like Teena, she asked me why I didn't tell her.

I told her for a few reasons, "I felt it was my fault, if I hadn't been drinking I wouldn't have been in that situation and if dad found out it would have ripped our family apart."

She understood my reasoning and we cried together. It was cleansing, and after we gathered ourselves we headed to the nursery. We have always had such a strong, unspoken bond between us that we never needed to mention the horror again. I will never reveal my secret to my father because the hurt would be unspeakable. I could convince my mother that she was not responsible, but my father would never understand. He would always feel that he could have done something to prevent it. I don't have to worry about him reading this book because his form of dyslexia makes it too difficult for him to read.

This is another example of how the twelve steps have helped me endure and progress. If it wasn't for all of those steps I wouldn't have been able to make peace with the man who raped me. I wouldn't have been able to forgive myself for the chaotic undertakings that ensued with my alcoholism and I wouldn't be here today, writing this book.

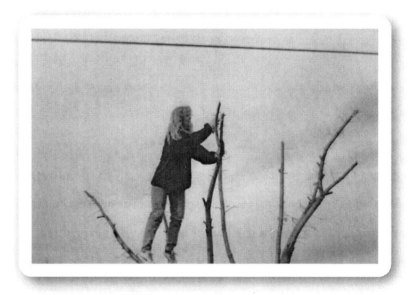

*Early sobriety, me finished pruning a tree.*

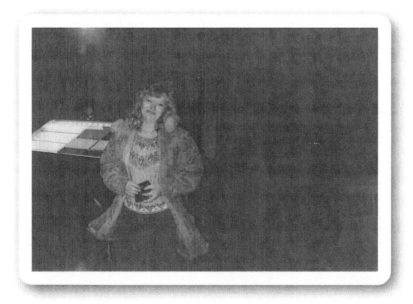

*Christmas shopping at the mall*

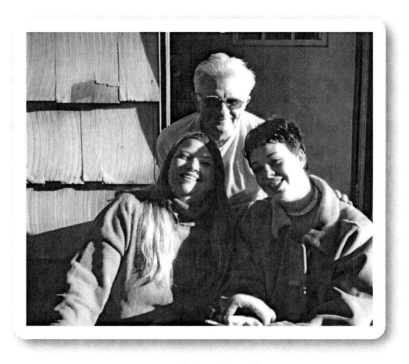

*Me, Ralph and Nicole*

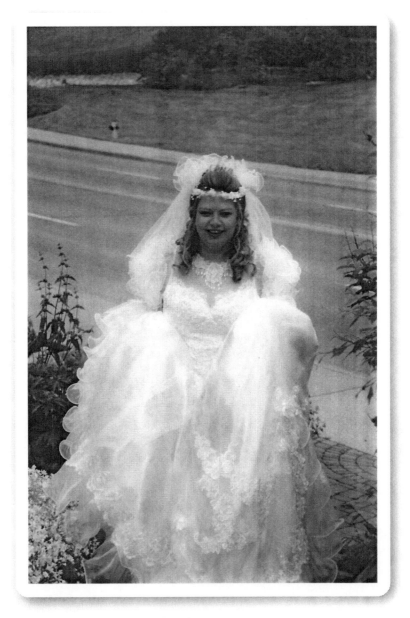

*Wedding day*

# The Crash

RALPH AND I MOVED IN TOGETHER AFTER MY MARRIAGE ENDED
with Tim. It wasn't long before I started slipping back into old
behaviours.

I began seeing a man named Troy that I worked with. When I first
met Troy I felt connected to him, this made me feel terrible because I
was still married to Tim. Troy and I had chemistry from the moment
we met. I felt more emotionally connected to Troy than I ever did
with Tim simply because we spent more time together. I never gave
Tim and I a chance because I was so consumed with what was right in
front of me. This was the main reason I ended our marriage, because
of the guilt I felt for connecting with and desiring Troy. I was having
an emotional affair.

After Tim and I separated, Troy and I's relationship progressed to
something legitimate. Troy looked like a bad boy, tough guy, the po-
lar opposite of Tim. I was attracted to him because he listened to me

gripe about my husband, when in reality I was griping about myself. I can see now that I was the problem in that marriage. Troy came across as a knight in shining armour saving his damsel in distress. Enabling the old behaviour I've been talking about, poor little victim Fiona.

Troy and I asked if we could get a load together so that we could bring my parents on the trip with us. We ended up getting dual loads to El Paso, my mother rode with me and my father rode with Troy. It was a holiday with my parents, whom didn't even know by this point that Troy and I were more than friends. It is also the last holiday I took with them. We had a beautiful time and I was elated I could bring my parents out of the country.

We were taking two loads of frozen meat [3]in bond to the Mexican border. When we arrived they took the meat from our trailers and unloaded it onto a dock in 110 degree weather. They just let it sit there, in the heat with the flies. For this reason, and this reason alone, if I ever travel to Mexico I will not eat the meat. My mother insisted I share this story with you. She was beside herself in shock when she witnessed it.

---

3    In Bond: A transportation provider U.S. Customs allows to carry customs-controlled merchandise between customs points. YRC Freight is a bonded carrier.

The rest of the trip we [4]deadheaded for 900 miles to California for two loads of bananas at Port Hueneme. On route we hit a terrible desert storm.

Harsh weather terrifies my poor mother, we were unable to see the road in front of us, dust and dirt were flying and we were forced to pull over. Once we could see past the sand we began driving again. My mother would have been happy to stay pulled over but we were already behind schedule.

Back on the road again, the lightening was outrageous, unlike anything I've ever witnessed before or after. Troy was driving in front of me and I could see the lightening cracking down all around us. A strike of lightening crashed near or on his trailer but it messed up the electronics in his trailer, making the lights flash erratically. My mother retreated to the bunk and did not return until we were parked in Yuma, Arizona. The storm was still present but had receded substantially, and it still took all three of us to convince her to leave the truck and get some dinner. I was happy I didn't mention the earthquake I experienced the last trip I took through that same route.

Troy wooed me with extravagant acts of kindness and professed his love in the slimiest but most romantic fashions. For example, one evening while we were freshly dating, I was on the phone with him

---

4      Deadhead: Deadhead is when a truck runs empty. After delivering a load, the truck won't pick another one up out of the same location. It will run empty to get to the next load.

just saying hello while he was in Vegas and on his way home. A few minutes later the doorbell rang and standing there, is Troy holding a dozen red roses, flashing his pretty boy smile. I was in the middle of dinner with Ralph and some girlfriends and they giggled and cooed ecstatically at his gesture. I was swept off my feet. I may sound a dash bitter writing this now, only because I know the outcome with this deceptive man.

Roughly six months into dating Troy and I moved in together. Troy got terminated from his position at our work and I foolishly followed him out the door. We went to work for another company out of Edmonton hauling flowers. This position required us to team drive, which meant, now we lived together and drove together. The reason we had to team drive flowers is because they are a hot commodity with a short life span. We spent every waking moment together. Let me tell you, you can learn a lot about a person by being that close for that long. Zero indiscretions which quickly lead to zero tolerance.

We were in Miami, FL and I was at the pool and running around on the grass. I was bitten by a fire ant and let me tell you, bug bites and I are a bad combination. My feet were burning so badly I spent the next four hours with my feet inside a toilet because it was the coldest water available.

On the road I had many encounters with insects which included a bite from a scorpion. I was bitten by a spider on the back of my knee which resulted in a substantial swelling and the loss of feeling in my leg. I was stung by a bee, which is how I discovered I am mildly allergic to bees. It sure baffled the nurse back in Calgary when I came in with an irritated bee sting in the middle of winter.

Troy was not the person he portrayed himself to be and I was guilty of the same crime. We both put our best foot forward, endearing each other in such a way we were ill prepared to meet the actual personalities behind our masks. After living with each other and then working with each other we both got to experience our less savoury sides. Our relationship lasted only a couple years and I'm happy that it ended because we brought out the worst in each other.

It wasn't long before Troy and I broke up. I found a different job that kept me busy and I was happy to focus on work. I had Moh and my truck and that was all I needed. I lived in my truck because I was literally always working. I had no time for relationships and I was happy for it, better for it. While on the road I had many opportunities to help a lot of folks, which in turn made me feel whole. Finally, I could give back for all that I had received over the years. I still attended meetings while I was on the road, the beauty of the program is that it's an international program and everyone is welcome from anywhere in the world.

One of the most awkward but also eye opening experiences was a meeting I attended in South Chicago. At this point I had a fairly sheltered life when it came to people of different ethnic backgrounds. I was the only fair skinned lady in the South Chicago meeting. I walked into that meeting feeling completely uncomfortable and overwhelmingly out of place. The man I had called prior to coming to the meeting walked up to me, he was 6'8" and just as intimidating as the whole group together.

I nervously offered a hand and he said, "We don't do that here sister."

I stood speechless and terrified. He reached down to me and gave me a big hug. I'm sure he must have felt the gasp of relief when I knew he wasn't going to harm me. They all welcomed me with open arms and it was one of the best meetings I have ever attended. I had never been put in a position of being a minority before or since that meeting and it was an awakening experience. Leaving that meeting I had the profound knowledge of empathy and unity.

Throughout the years and the vast miles I travelled I made many lifelong friends. I practiced the twelve steps with devotion and even got to help others on twelve step calls as I was helped in Texas that first time. I learned a lot about others, which was remarkable because I came from a long line of selfish behaviour. I got to peer into the souls of different people and they were all as painstakingly human as I was. Looking for the same things I desired, to be heard and loved. So I offered them an ear and my empathy and that sufficed.

In 2003 I changed jobs again. I started work with Jayco International and rented a little basement suite in Calgary.

One day my mother came on a run with me, we were stopped by the Mexican border, waiting 22 hours for a single skid of lettuce. This is a completely normal procedure for a trucker. As we sat waiting, we saw another female driver who was waiting for her load as well. She was making rounds going from truck to truck and my mom couldn't understand what on earth she was doing, going in and out of all these trucks.

"What is she doing?" my mother exclaimed baffled.

"Well mom, she has a part time job" I snickered.

"What do you mean?" she was still puzzled.

"Well, she has a full time job trucking, but on her down time she has a part time job" I emphasized but she was still perplexed. "She's a lot lizard" I stated.

"What on earth is that?"

"A lot lizard is someone who performs sexual favours for money."

My mother's jaw dropped, she sat completely speechless while I giggled in the corner.

In later years my father would ask me jokingly, "What are you doing wasting your time sitting around on that money-maker?" which still makes me chuckle to this day.

A week before May long weekend in 2005 my uncle Charlie passed away while I was in Arizona. Uncle Charlie was the closest man my father had to his own father. I was beside myself when I heard the news. I loaded up my truck and drove straight for Calgary in a daze. Trying to focus on getting home, I hadn't completed my log book for two days and I was pulled over just outside of Flagstaff, AZ. The officer was really nice to me and when I told him about my uncle's passing he let me off without so much as a ticket. I'm not sure exactly how I made it back to Calgary because the entire trip is a blur. But I did make it back, safe and sound.

The funeral was scheduled for a Thursday afternoon and I made it home Thursday evening. Exhausted, I was devastated that I had missed paying my last respects to dear old Uncle Charlie. They couldn't have held the funeral off any longer either because of a rodeo that was taking place May long weekend.

I dropped my truck off at the yard, went straight home and crashed. I was awake again at midnight because I had to deliver my load for 3am.

It was 1:30am and I was driving down 84th Street, it was a pitch black night, the moon nowhere to be seen. As I was nearing my turn, I put on my blinker and slowed. I was clear to turn into the yard. Before making my turn I looked into the rear-view mirror once more, at that moment I knew things would never be the same again.

I could see headlights and I knew by the way they were barreling down on me that they were going way too fast. It was instinctual and I could feel that they didn't know that I was there.

I made a split-second decision that probably saved my life. I swung into the oncoming lane, opposite from where I was turning, luckily the street was vacant.

The impact of the crash was petrifying as I was shot seventy five feet into the ditch. I was hit by a '78 Malibu going 140 km/hr.

This singular incident impacted my life on so many levels, defining the remainder of my life.

While in the ditch, my initial reaction was fear approaching almost immediate anger. Moh and I were in my truck being told not to move by some gentleman who had stopped and was now standing outside my door. He had been driving a truck pulling a 'super B trailer when he came across my wreck. I wish to this day I knew who he was because he was like a guardian angel. We watched as the man who hit me was trying to get out of his car on the other side of the road. In that moment I realised why he hit me. He was so intoxicated that when he opened his door he fell right into the street.

It was not long before emergency response vehicles arrived and people were milling around. The rest of this night is spotty at best but there are many painful pieces still prominent within my memory.

Paramedics and firemen were at the side of my truck talking to me through my window. They couldn't get me out because the door was jammed shut.

I remember someone asking if the dog would bite. I said no.

They were understandably uncertain considering the circumstances.

Somehow they ended up getting the door open. I had to remain in

---

5    Two trailers linked together by a fifth wheel, and are up to 26 m (85 ft) long.

my seat until someone looked me over before I could climb out. I sat in shock while someone coaxed Moh out of the truck. I was far more concerned for Moh's welfare than my own and I distinctly remember the immediate pain felt by her absence as they took her away from me. I was terrified I would lose her.

They pulled me out of my truck after attaching a neck brace. Now I was seething. When I saw the man who hit me the adrenaline took over and I completely lost it. The policemen had to hold me back as I was lunging for him. I wanted to kill him.

I was screaming at the top of my lungs, "WHAT KIND OF IDIOT ARE YOU? HOW DARE YOU DO THIS!"

Looking back I was ranting like a crazy lady. I wouldn't have killed him if I had been able to break free from those officers. I'm pretty certain I would have kicked him in his family jewels though.

So there I was, being all disruptive and disagreeable on the side of the road while this drunk driver was too sloshed to care.

My disagreeing didn't stop in the ditch either; I also refused to go to the hospital.

I told the officers quite plainly, "I have work to do."

After all, I was right at the corner of the yard where my semi was parked with a full load of produce that needed to be delivered at 3. I really did have work to do. If that isn't a statement of my work ethic, I'm not sure what is.

The officer looked at me with sad eyes and said, "That is not happening. Is there anyone you can call?"

By this point I was a bit fearful. I realized that it was already past 2:30. I called my dispatcher, Kevin, who had been sleeping and spoke with him quickly.

The officer took the phone away from me as I was saying, "I'm going to head home."

I guess they felt that I shouldn't be making anymore irrational decisions.

I waited for someone, anyone to take me home. By this time the drunken man was gone by ambulance to the hospital. I was still refusing an ambulance so the police had to succumb to my terms and find a way to trick me into going to the hospital.

My boss arrived and took my load to its delivery after checking in on me. My friend had also been called to pick up Moh.

I was certain the police were just going to take me home to rest but they didn't, lying buggers.

The two kind police officers put me into the back of their SUV and off we went. We chatted along the way and it didn't take me too long to realize something was up when we passed the corner that would take me home.

"Where are we going?" I asked with a smidgen of attitude.

They smiled kindly at me and continued to drive. I should have known something was up when they had me all bundled in blankets. As I look back now, it's a little easier to put the pieces together.

We arrived at the hospital where they boarded me onto a stretcher. I was hazy of what was happening around me and for some reason, my memories are not near as vivid as at the crash site. I'm sure being highly medicated had something to do with this.

My next conscious memory was around 7am when they let me talk to Kevin, who had called to check on me. He was seeing if I would be ready to head out by noon, he had a load for me going to Ohio. I said, of course I would be good to go.

The nurses overheard this little exchange and I was informed that I would not be able to make it in for my load to Ohio. I had been given medication through the early morning hours that restricted me from driving.

I was shaking so badly that I spilled water I was attempting to drink down the front of my very flattering hospital garb. If I had known then, what I know now, I would have fallen madly in love with this attire. There were many years to follow after this incident where I would be sporting it.

Kevin said, "Fiona, I've called your folks, they are heading over there now."

I discovered that as a truck driver, you never want your family called at six in the morning. Kevin had called my folks and when the caller ID showed the name of my work, my parents feared the worst. It is never a call you want to answer as a parent, child or spouse of a driver.

The hospital released me at noon and although I was shaking less, I was still shaking. My parents drove me home where Kevin and his wife were waiting for me. My parents were unable to come in because the basement suite I lived in was not wheelchair accessible. Pearl, Kevin's wife, promised my mother that they would take good care of me. They sure did.

Pearl and Kevin got me down into my suite. There was already a beautiful bouquet of flowers on my kitchen table from them.

Feeling incredibly sore following the accident, I was booked off work to recover. I spent a lot of time on my couch. Being booked off work to recover might have been okay if I had been getting paid for it, but the moment my body ceased so did my income. I was a sub-contractor with no insurance. All I had was benefits for prescriptions, and even though I had been paying into workers compensation, because that bastard hit me on my way to work and not while I was at work I did not qualify. So now, I was crippled from the accident, out of work, receiving $1200 a month from my car insurance with no other income coming in and expenses piling up.

I started going to therapy for post-traumatic stress disorder (PTSD). Throughout my sessions I would soon discover that PTSD was the least of my problems.

A plethora of issues arose.

I had terrible anxiety about driving, even sitting in a passenger seat made me sketchy. I lost all faith in all other drivers, terrified of being in another collision.

I had incredibly low self-esteem with high expectations of myself which only made it impossible to attain any confidence at all. I battled greatly with my loss of independence, I felt completely useless and this bruised my ego worse than the physical pain from the crash.

My therapist recognized that I was overshadowing my fear and anxiety with humour, trying to make light of my situation even though I was utterly terrified of losing myself completely.

Not much time after the accident I received an eviction notice from my landlord, this really amplified my anxiety. I was asked to move because my landlord was perfectly comfortable renting the illegal suite to someone who was barely home. But now that I was stuck at home they became annoyed. I needed people to assist me in my day to day activities, after the eviction, the situation became quite uncomfortable while I had to search for a new home. I had to find one without stairs because they were becoming unbearable to climb.

I had many people assist me during this period, including Bone and his girlfriend. I remember requiring him to help me out of the shower because my body was just too sore. It was embarrassing, although I was very grateful, I was also mortified. I had always viewed him as my son and now, before being close to a ripe old age, I needed his assistance just to get out of the tub.

This was a drastic change from what I was used to, my independence had been snatched away with my health on the fateful night of the crash.

I found out that the man who hit me was not driving his own car; it belonged to someone who didn't live in the province. This meant that the drunk was not insured, which would become a whole other ball of wax.

I began dating a man that I had known for a long time from the program named Craig. I was serving coffee during a meeting and just like Ruby, he asked me out.

His exact words were, "If you ever quit smoking, I'd do you in a heartbeat."

I found it funny and I called him a pig, then we went for a walk in the park.

Things gradually progressed into a romance, he was sweet and caring and courteous. This was exactly what I needed at the time.

Various symptoms were starting to occur including feelings of numbness in my limbs and short term memory loss.

July 1, 2005 I rented a main floor of a house with a kind landlord. There were two extra rooms and I was given permission to sublet them as a means to assist with my circumstances. Craig moved me into the new house and our relationship blossomed from there.

Craig was always put off by my health and the circumstances surrounding it, but he still stuck around and rooted me on as I regained my strength.

I was attending physio and acupuncture three times a week, luckily my insurance covered it. I traded in the keys for my truck for a job in the office of my work. This turned out to be quite hard on me emotionally. I would be billing and going through invoices, seeing where all the loads were going and coming from. It broke my heart to know that I was missing out on so much already.

I was very much in denial of my physical limitations. I still imagined that I would return to my old life one day. Like that was possible.

Working in the office I was constantly staring at a computer screen and I noticed my vision started going a little wonky. Then at physio, I was staring at a metal towel warming chamber with words inscribed in blue across it. With a blink, the blue disappeared and the color was gone. It scared me and I informed my physio therapist who found it just as strange and concerning.

My vision continued to falter and by the next session, the left side of my body weakened and almost stopped functioning altogether. I was immediately taken to a hospital, fearful I had suffered a stroke. At the hospital they performed a [6]CAT scan which came out unremarkable with no anomalies.

Not long after I fell down my stairs and lost consciousness temporarily. I had no idea how this occurred and no recollection of the fall, all I remembered was waking up.

---

6    Also known as CT, it is a special X-ray test that produces cross-sectional images of the body using X-rays and a computer.

I was booked for an [7]MRI and taken off computer work from then on. While I waited for the results of the MRI, my health steadily declined. I had to start using a walker for the first time in my life, this really bruised my pride. My father, my grandfather and Craig built a ramp at the entrance of my home so I could wheel my walker into my house.

No longer driving, I was taking a bus downtown to board a [8]C-Train over to a Southside station where my boss, Jim, would pick me up and take me to the office. I would complete the paperwork in my sad state of dismay wondering how my life had fallen out of my hands so quickly. The office gave me jobs that catered the best to my new restrictions, it was a nice gesture.

In October 2005, around the time of my birthday, I was called into the doctor's office to receive test results.

The MRI showed anomalies. The report showed 16 lesions on my brain.

The doctor looked at me and said, "I'm sorry to tell you this but I have to book you into the Multiple Sclerosis clinic. There's nothing I can do for you."

---

7    Magnetic resonance imaging is a noninvasive medical test that helps physicians diagnose and treat medical conditions. It uses a powerful magnetic field, radio frequency pulses and a computer to produce detailed pictures of organs, soft tissues, bone and virtually all other internal body structures.

8    C-Train is the light rail transit (LRT) system in Calgary, Alberta, Canada

My initial reaction was anger because of how nonchalant he had just delivered this devastating news. I couldn't believe he held no shred of empathy for me. I didn't understand that he was just a doctor doing his job.

Because of the lengthy history of MS within my family it was not a shock when they found out. It was disheartening, but not a shock, it certainly didn't make it any easier.

All I could think was, "Happy effing birthday to me."

Craig reacted okay and told me that he would be there for me to the best of his abilities. From that point on he never attended a doctor's appointment or participated in anything to do with my health.

This was my first revelation that he was not okay with my disease.

My first appointment at the MS clinic was in November and I felt somewhat relieved. Relieved I had confirmation that all of the things that were going wrong inside my body were real. I had expressed concerns of my health in recovery meetings before I was diagnosed with MS and they were kyboshed. People were trying to convince me that my health issues were all in my head and that I was merely seeking attention.

Now, after much time, I could finally move forward and start treatment to get myself better. All over again, only this time it was with MS and not alcoholism.

In December I received results from another MRI, the 16 lesions grew to 19. The progression of my disease was exponential from the onset. To have three new lesions in two months was terribly remarkable.

I went back to work just after Christmas, back to driving my beloved truck.

I was not ready to go back to work, but the doctor that worked for my car insurance company stated that my MS was not a result of the crash and therefore could no longer be covered. I had no choice but to continue to work that or starve.

Before they let me return to driving I had to do a road trip with my boss in the passenger seat confirming I could handle the job. I did fine, but I knew in my heart I was not fine. I could not bring Moh with me so she moved in with my parents. She had been injured badly as well in the crash and could no longer jump into the truck. So there I was, doing the job I loved, not feeling good about it and without my companion.

I spoke at a MADD meeting to tell my story of the heartbreak my experience caused. It was therapeutic to be able to share my story and caution others.

At the time I had a [9]'sponsee' that was the perpetrator in a drunken driving incident which resulted in the death of a mother. She was supposed to speak with me, but she was not ready to face that kind

---

9    'Sponsee' is a reference I use for the people I sponsor in the 12 step program.

of confrontation. She helped me as much as I helped her, perhaps more because she taught me forgiveness and redemption on levels I couldn't fathom prior.

Days turned into months and I was feeling unwell the whole time. One evening while attending a meeting, a friend insisted I go to a hospital because I looked so ill.

My first hospitalization was for a severe kidney infection. I was hospitalized for two weeks. I was throwing up constantly. The nurse would bring me a pan to vomit into because I didn't have the energy to make it to the toilet.

The nurses were so horrible that they never changed or emptied my vomit pan.

When I received my meal trays, the staff would place it right next to the foul bowl. I put in a complaint with the hospital because the care was so appalling.

On April 12, 2006 I had to put my dear Moh down. The damage was too severe and almost a year later she had succumbed to her injuries. Her hips were damaged badly and she couldn't even jump into a minivan. I could no longer watch her struggle and suffer so when I saw that her condition was not getting any better I made the difficult choice to put her down and out of her misery. This broke my already aching heart into a thousand pieces.

I was in denial of how quickly my disease was progressing and as a result I had many learning curves. My bladder and bowels were failing and I had to buy pull-ups. However, because of my pride I did not put them on and suffered the consequences of incontinence in public.

On day I was at a truck stop in Jerome, Idaho. I was parked in a handicap stall where I had made it to the bathroom in time before soiling myself, I was elated. I got up after I was finished and headed to my truck. About ten feet outside the door I could feel my bowels starting to function again. I was closer to the bathroom than my truck so I headed back inside. As soon as I stepped inside I could feel my bowels release. Excrement dripped down my legs, through my pants, onto my shoes and then to the floor. I kept walking to the bathroom with my head down, leaving a poop trail the whole way. I walked into the handicap stall, closed the door, took my pants off and began weeping uncontrollably.

I heard a dainty voice say, "hello," from behind the door and then she said, "Is there anything I can do to help you?"

"If you don't mind there is," I said through my tears, "Here's the key to my truck," I threw the key under the stall door, "my truck is parked in the handicap stall outside."

"What do you need me to do?" she asked.

"When you get in my truck, can you snoop through the drawers and find me some pants and behind my driver's seat there is a bag of pull-ups."

I heard her giggle from behind the door which made me laugh with her. She immediately saw the silliness in my behaviour and now

I could too.

She brought me diapers and clean pants and it was one of the nicest things anyone has ever done for me. She was such a kind soul to help me out while I was in my moment of despair. I pushed my grief aside and cleaned myself up, discarding my soiled clothing. When I exited the restroom there was a staff member mopping up my mess. Nobody said anything, they simply smiled and carried on and I was grateful.

You'd think after all of that humiliation I would start wearing my damn pull-ups. But I was convinced that this was just a slip up and I still had control of my disease.

I had many more accidents to follow.

I was supposed to be using a cane to assist my walking and I stubbornly didn't which led me to fall numerous times. Within the course of six months I had lost my wallet three times in the US. Thank God my work held records of my identification otherwise I wouldn't have been able to get back into my own country.

The first six months was enlightening, not only for learning how to work with my disease but also how the people in my life changed and left. Some I grew closer with, while others couldn't cope with watching their quickly deteriorating friend.

Craig was someone who drifted further away. I tried to shelter my disease from him for fear he would leave. I did so by working hard throughout my shift and then resting the entire way home so that I could recover enough to make dinner or make love with him that evening. I tried to convince him and myself I wasn't as sick as I really was.

In the spring of 2006 I started taking [10]Copaxone which is a daily injection to minimize MS flare ups. I had to rotate injections in five different locations on my body, my hip, arm, stomach, thigh or buttocks. I always injected into my stomach because it was the least painful site. If I injected into my thighs my legs would immediately go into spasms. It was very painful and I avoided doing this at all costs.

I continued to work and then the government was on my ass for my taxes I hadn't filed. As a subcontractor I had saved $14,000 to pay my dues, but I ended up needing the money. I used it for the time I was forced to take off work after my accident. This money quickly became a means for survival. I only received enough money each month from my insurance to cover my rent, and my new car I couldn't drive.

Please keep in mind that because of my upbringing I refused and still have never sought (let alone received) government assistance. After watching all the trouble my parents had with Assisted Income for the Severely Handicapped (AISH) I had no desire to put myself in

---

10      Copaxone: is a synthetic protein made up of a combination of four amino acids that chemically resemble a component of myelin (the insulating material that protects nerves and helps them work properly). Copaxone induces the production of immune cells that are less damaging to myelin. Definition from http://mssociety.ca/en/treatments/modify_copaxone.htm

that position.

So now I owed the government $14,000 in unpaid taxes which I had originally saved but depleted over the course of nine months to sustain. I worked out a payment plan with them that I would pay $250 per month until the debt was balanced. On top of this I owed $16,000 for GST and if that wasn't paid I would have faced jail time. Reluctantly, I asked my parents to help me out and they did by taking out a loan. I felt like such a burden having to ask them for this substantial amount of money when they were barely scraping by themselves.

Everything was going downhill at an incredibly fast pace. I was falling down constantly, imbalanced with severe incontinence and my medication was not working. I was still driving long haul, full time, only coming home one evening every week. I exhausted myself trying to pay my debts.

One day Bone showed up at my house with a friend of ours, Jason, who had been sober for seven years. Jason was relapsing, homeless, hung-over and sick when they walked in the door. I fed them and they stayed the day, I also had a few more guests including a sponsee who had just given me $250 cash as a gift that I had put in my wallet. Jason stole my laptop and my wallet after I invited him into my home and filled his belly with a home cooked meal.

I was beside myself with his behavior. It was the epitome of an addict and an ultimate low to steal from someone who offered all they could while struggling themselves.

I was losing faith in humanity and in myself, exhausted all the time. My hopes that I would get better were fading. My MS was overtaking my body and my mind, weakening them and I was becoming conflicted with faith in my own abilities.

I attempted to quit my job, surrendering to my symptoms. I just didn't feel competent and it was both excruciating and exhausting. My work persuaded me to stay through promises of working better with my health. They held up their end of this deal.

If you had told me that things were about to get worse, I would have laughed in your face. I was merely at the top of a steep hill of bad health and suffering.

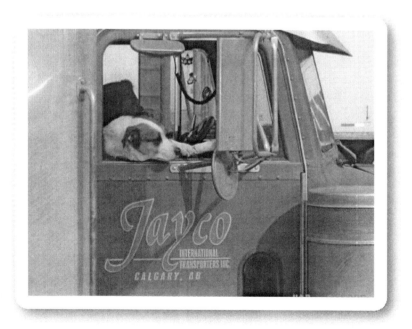

*Moh sitting in my truck*

# Denial & Changes

MOST OF 2007 WAS AN ERRATIC AND HECTIC YEAR. I FILED A LAW-suit against the drunk driver and the owner of the car because the drunk driver had no insurance. I learned that the moment your keys are in someone else's hands, you are 100% liable. Poor luck for the fellow who lent his car out to the drunken buffoon who hit me.

I was still working full time and taking two days off every week. In those two days I would cram in several appointments. I worked my ass off trying to pay my immense debt to the government.

I was clinging to the hope that I could salvage my old life. I was bitter with the man who had hit me, triggering my disease. I was bitter in meetings because I was listening to stories from drunk drivers and when some would try to justify their behaviour it made me want to ring their necks. I was sitting there crippled from a drunken driving accident while people bragged about getting off their charges because they had decent legal counsel. Feeling quite sensitive, I found myself dwelling on my disabilities, unable to find solace. When a MADD commercial came on the television my blood would boil. I had people approaching me constantly, telling me they knew about the next new miracle cure for my disease. Suddenly, everyone had PhD and I was maxing out my credit card, incurring more debt trying to save myself by purchasing these 'miraculous cures'.

My parents were devastated having to watch their daughter flail. I was like a bird caught in a windstorm of my newfound disease and I couldn't keep my grips. I would visit them on my days off, and they always looked happy to see me, but beneath the surface I could sense the fear.

I had been in search for an accountant for some time. I would have never been in the big mess with the government I was if I had one to begin with. Luckily, I met a wonderful woman named Cecile through an office I had inquired about my circumstances. Cecile knew that working with me would not be easy, I didn't have a lot to offer her but she helped me anyway.

I brought in a ton of boxes filled with slips and receipts, a chaotic mess. She sifted through each box, one by one, organizing all my finances. She was a gift from the heavens because I know that nobody else would have ever done what she has done for me.

I should have claimed bankruptcy well before this time, but my pride and my ego would not allow me. Now I feel foolish about it because I could have saved myself a lot of money. I just had to pay my debts, whether I could afford it or not. I suffered more so I could pay them, completely self-inflicted as usual.

Craig moved in and we were content, both too busy to have any real issues. The sex was phenomenal and when I think about it now, the sex was all that really kept us together. We didn't have many opportunities to spend time together, but when we did it was between the sheets.

My MS was always considered active and because of this I qualified for full funding for my medications. I was fortunate because they totalled just over $7000 each month. After they realized the Copaxone was having no effect, I stopped taking the injections for three months so I could start a Disease Modifying Drug (DMD). At this time the only DMD medications for MS they had were injections, there were no oral medications available. The only treatment for this disease at that time was incredibly painful.

One of my first revelations with my MS symptoms was the nerves in my central nervous system. Every time I would bow my head I would feel these tiny electrical charges shoot out my feet. I used to call them my foot orgasms because they tickled and made me giggle every time. It made me look like a mad woman to many I'm sure, but I thought it was a riot.

Work required me to visit the US Department of Agriculture (USDA) once a week. I made good friends with the boys that worked there, we just jived.

One day I was telling them about these foot orgasms, "If I could get these suckers to come out the right body part or bottle them and sell them, I could retire tomorrow"

From that moment on they referred to me as Sparky. So if you ever happen to go by the USDA, tell them Sparky says hi.

I brought it up to the doctor, and she didn't concur with my reaction. Talk about putting a damper on your day. I finally find an amusing aspect of this damned disease and it's 'inappropriate'. Thanks a lot.

Not long after, I started becoming very heat sensitive. I'm not sure if it was the heat sensitivity per say that started all of it, but I had an incident while driving through Southern Colorado into Northern New Mexico. It was scorching and I had been doing everything in my power to relieve myself from the heat.

The entire left side of my body had gone completely numb, like a dentist had snuck in and injected Novocaine into my body parts. I was numb from my left knee all the way to the left side of my waist. I continued to drive and suddenly I had a feeling, like something crawled across my pelvis, grabbed the numbness and pulled it over to the right side numbing everything in between my knees and waist. Like when your limbs fall asleep, it tickled because the nerves were alive and active. I continued to drive because I was already getting used to these little oddities. I was aware it was my nerves but it was all still very foreign to me. I believe that the heat was the cause of this particular reaction. To this day, my sensation is still completely out of order.

My bitterness made me stop attending meetings for a while. I just didn't have the patience to listen to people who complained about things that seemed menial to me. I was experiencing this colossal, life altering ailment and they were complaining about a rude passenger on the bus. I was utterly intolerant to listening to one more person complain about their 'bad day'. Thankfully I was still able to hang around with the people who tolerated my self-pity.

One day a good friend of mine said, "Fiona, have you ever driven drunk?"

I was appalled by this question because I knew I had. I had been bitching for months about drunken drivers. "Well yes" I said defensively.

"Well be honest with yourself, it could have just as easily been you who did the same to someone else." He was being blunt, telling me exactly what I needed to hear and I was furious.

I knew that he was right and I didn't want to admit it, I left in a huff and wallowed in more self-pity for a few days before really considering the facts.

In a way he saved me from myself, he was a good friend for telling me what he knew I needed but didn't want to hear. Needless to say, I stopped bitching about drunk drivers. I completed a step five and regained awareness once more of my own being. It never occurred to me to complete a step five with my disease, I was pretty sure I could manage this bump in the road. I was convinced that my disease was all in my head and I just needed to ignore it and eventually it would go away.

Even though I wasn't attending meetings I still kept up with my duties as a sponsor and sponsee. I enjoyed helping others because it was a chance for me to get out of my own head. Yet I had sponsee's dropping me because they didn't want to burden me with their problems and this made me sad.

There were a couple of women who took it upon themselves to bad mouth me and degrade my illness. They were sure that I was embellishing most of my symptoms because they weren't typical for my disease. It infuriated me that people were listening to them and I had no way of proving to them that what I was experiencing was real.

I discovered hard truths about the people around me that I believed were my friends. They would talk about me behind my back and ridicule my incontinence, all of this would be revealed to me by my real friends.

There were friends I had for so long, I didn't want to believe they could be so cruel, surely our friendship meant more. Sadly, I was wrong. It really affected me in a way that made me cynical and untrusting. Even to this day I have a hard time trusting people. My supposed friends had downgraded my illness so often that I started questioning myself too and still sometimes do.

I was in a whirlwind of health ailments, untrue friendships, massive debt riding on my shoulders, suffering from a disease where symptoms are triggered by stress. It was no wonder I was on the steady decline. It was absolute lunacy and I felt alone. I still have some very loyal people but my cynical side was overwhelming and taking over my thoughts. I could only focus on who and what I didn't have in my life. I couldn't shake the feeling that I desperately needed all that I had lost. At that time, the hurt outweighed the good.

There is one person in particular that I would love to confront but I have never had the opportunity. Perhaps she bothers me because there are so many others like her, but here is an example of the betrayal of trust from my so-called friend, Daisy.

I met Daisy at a meeting and there's something about her that I was always aware of but chose to accept anyways. She was a fair-weather friend. It's pretty self-explanatory but if you don't know what a fair-weather friend is, it is a friend who stops being a friend when there are hard times. I've had a lot of these friends but for some reason, Daisy stands out. Maybe it's because Ruby had an affair with her years before, but she also said many hurtful things about me at a time when I trusted and needed her friendship.

She would say things like, "Fiona isn't that sick, she's exaggerating" she would ridicule my 'accidents' to my friends. She found a lot of entertainment by stabbing me in the back; the worst part is there were so many others who joined in too.

I had stopped therapy by this point because I had no time. In reality I was running away. I filled my timetable with work, attempting to pay back my debt to no avail. Each month I was making payments to the government of $250 while incurring $1000 in penalties and interest. I was chasing my tail and the stress was relentless making my body shut down.

I horribly lied about my health to Craig and he seemed content while I was doing that. I was seeing the doctors at the MS clinic every 3-6 months while most patients only have appointments once a year. This factor alone should have been a red flag but I was still in denial.

I love the MS clinic. I had a nurse named Kathy who was such a treasure. She's an angel, unanimously loved because her soul is so pure. She was always honest about everything which is exactly what I needed, even though I hardly listened. She was constantly trying to bring me back to reality, patient and subtle as she was. With the exception of one doctor, I've always been treated with great dignity and respect at the MS clinic. They were concerned about my lifestyle and my denial, but they were patient and respected my courage and strength. I'm a determined, strong and resilient woman when it comes to MS and they recognized that – even through my stubborn tendencies.

One day I was in Red Deer hooking up to a trailer. I was walking in my sandals and somehow cut my big toe. I had been having sensory issues before this, especially in my feet and I had no clue that I was even hurt. I walked into the security shack to sign paperwork and the woman behind the counter just about had a coronary.

She dialed 911 while grabbing the first aid kit saying, "Fiona! You need to sit down, there's a pool of blood around your foot and it's increasing by the second!"

I looked down bewildered and could see she was even more baffled because I had no idea. An ambulance arrived and cleaned me up, I was lucky I didn't need stitches but the paramedics were concerned because I hadn't felt the injury. When I told them I had MS they seemed more understanding. This kind of stuff was becoming pretty regular and I was still oblivious about the severity of my disease.

Nobody can tell Fiona how quick she is.

It got to the point where I was no longer able to drive within the city because it was becoming increasingly uncomfortable to drive in major metropolises. I began manipulating my schedule as a means to avoid heavy traffic.

My left leg was becoming very weak and it was difficult to keep my foot on the clutch for extended periods. I sucked up my pride and decided to look for work elsewhere that didn't require me to use my left leg and would hopefully be easier in general. I also had to change vehicles because it became difficult to drive a standard; I purchased a 2002 automatic Sebring with a speed stick so I could still have the illusion of driving manually.

Getting the new job was a difficult process. Believe it or not, not a lot of people want to hire a sick person. The interviews would go well until I would say I had MS and then they'd ask me why I was changing jobs.

I would tell them honestly, "My left leg doesn't work. I need a truck without a clutch."

I only applied with companies who had automatic trucks for that very specific reason. Constantly, I was undermined and asked why I would waste my time when no one in their right mind would hire the likes of me. I didn't give up though; just because my leg was giving me issues did not make me any less of a great driver. I just needed to modify. I also needed someone to give me the chance.

After half a year of searching I finally found a new job with an amazing company that supplied me with an automatic truck as well as a terrific dispatcher named Larry. Larry worked with my needs from day one.

A prime example of how amazing Larry is, one day I was in Ontario, CA. I phoned him to refuse a load that was waiting for me. I couldn't pick it up because when I awoke my nerves were stabbing me with what felt like ice picks into my knuckles. I couldn't steer, let alone open my hands. He made arrangements booking me off for two days without a fuss or a question. He did this sort of thing for me whenever I needed and it helped me be honest with myself about my condition. I was always more honest with my work than I was with my doctors about my symptoms.

One April afternoon in 2008, while working with my new company I arrived at a yard outside of Taber, AB for a load of French fries. It was the weekend so there was nobody around when I went to hook up my trailer. They had dropped the trailer off on a concrete pad and the hook up point was mere inches from the edge of the concrete. I was trying to hook the trailer up while avoiding a pool of freezing water that had gathered at the surface.

I was avoiding the water because I am incredibly sensitive to it, the colder the water, the more excruciatingly scorching it feels to me. It feels like I am being burnt continuously with matches.

I was grasping the bottom of the trailer while crab walking along the small strip of pavement so I didn't have to get my feet wet. I got to the dolly handle while still in my crab stance and began retracting the dolly legs. My legs gave out and I smoked my head against the side of the trailer, knocking myself out cold and landing right into the puddle I had tried so hard to avoid. If my lower body had landed in that puddle I may have woken up sooner but thankfully only upper body did which isn't too partial to the burning pain caused by cool water.

I woke a couple hours later with a terrible headache. After crawling under the trailer, still trying to avoid getting my legs wet, I gathered myself, put on a fresh change of clothing and continued to work.

This was one of my worst experiences endured while working.

My medication doses were getting higher and higher. I was maxing out on dosages for my nerve pain meds, my muscles relaxants and several others. The side effects would have incapacitated a grown man but I continued to work. I would drive all day, seven days a week until I ran out of hours. In North America, driving 70 hours in eight days is the legal limit.

I was learning to manage the medication by being in touch with my body. I was able to tweak the dosages for my own comfort, with minimal side effects while still effectively treating my symptoms. Not a lot of people are aware that they can take this kind of initiative; they feel they have to follow their doctors' recommendations until they are dope-stupid. I believe the doctors need the patient's feedback or preference to successfully treat anyone. I could not, nor will not tolerate succumbing to being doped up. This is why I was able to work effectively while enduring the many issues and symptoms arising from my MS.

Moving along, I have learned how to micro manage my medications. I'm still working, in denial but subconsciously becoming more aware, trying to pay off my debts and disguise the severity of my disease to my boyfriend.

I bought a house in Coleman, AB in the Crowsnest Pass in May '09. By buying the house I had acquired an asset that the government could take away. I hoped this would make them get off my ass a little bit. Let me tell you, that plan worked. I also bought the house because I wanted to own something.

My mother used to tell me that, "If you own dirt, the world opens up to you."

So I bought dirt with a house on top of it and Craig and I moved in. Funny thing, I ended up finding the wallet that held the $250 gifted to me under my sink. I found it while I was packing to move to Coleman, Jason had clearly taken the money and stashed the wallet there.

When we moved I realized how nice it was to escape the city. I was brought back to reality of what I was really missing out on. Craig quit his job when we moved, assuming he could find a job in the mines close by. This was not so. I knew it would be difficult for him, I tried to encourage him to find work before we moved but he was convinced it wouldn't be a problem. He ended up unemployed and all the financial responsibilities landed in my lap. This was very exhausting and stressful, which ignited my symptoms.

I was working so much that I was only taking 36 hours off just so I could reset my log book and get back to working. I was constantly getting urinary tract infections (UTI), Craig started anti-depressants and our sex life was non-existent. Our only connection was now in the gutter.

The passion was fading and fear started taking over. I was sicker than I had ever been by this point, falling down constantly, the muscles in my legs were giving out and my balance was completely off. I was tripping over my own feet and landing on my face in the dirt or on the pavement. My incontinence was worsening; I was wearing diapers all the time, hardly ever able to make it to a toilet in time. As soon as I stood up, my bladder or bowels would release and I had absolutely no control. No matter how many times I soil myself, even to this day, it always makes me feel melancholic. It's something I can never get used to and it's a terrible bruise on my dignity.

I ended up on short term disability because my symptoms were becoming so severe. I was having really bad spasms in the back of my right leg that would shoot from my knee, down my calf and into my ankle. I could no longer drive.

I had to be off work with no pay for two weeks before short term disability would take effect. So now Craig and I were both unemployed and for two weeks, we had zero income coming in. We were not getting along and I was searching for anything that might bring some peace into our lives.

Craig's seventeen year old daughter, Nicole, came up for a visit from Iowa in the fall. Craig hadn't seen her in a decade and I thought she could bring the peace I so desperately desired. To this day, I classify her as my own daughter and am currently a Nana to her child. I set up and paid for the visit in an attempt to console Craig, hoping this would make him feel better. It was wonderful for me to meet his beautiful child and accept her as my own. She would end up becoming the only child I never had.

She stayed for a few weeks and reconnected with Craig while I connected with her. I changed her life during that visit, she arrived as a rebel without a clue, and by the time she left she had gained a new perspective. She returned home, improved her grades and graduated, and went to college. She is now a Certified Nursing Assistant (CNA).

At the time I didn't know I had influenced her to make such wonderful achievements, she later confessed to me her motivation through one of our many conversations.

I think the inspiration for her pursuing a line of work that helped others was from our first visit. She would watch me fall down and pick myself back up and then watch her father's reaction to it all.

Nicole would jump to help me up and Craig would bark at her, "sit down and leave her alone, she can get up by herself."

I'm not sure if Craig reacted this way as a means to make me stronger and more independent, but there were many times I could have used his support. I don't believe his intentions were ever bad. It was just his funny way of coping with my disease. By the third week of October, Nicole had left to go back to Iowa and Craig started working part time at a ski shop in Calgary, fixing skis. He was a ski bum, and worked more for the perks than the money. His selfishness was more visible than ever when it came to skis. He spent more time in the shop than he ever spent with me during the winter months.

I was still on disability and barely able to care for myself. I was getting sicker by the day, stuck alone in a town where I knew nobody. If it weren't for my friends I met in recovery I likely would have died. There were a few people I knew from Calgary that resided in Crowsnest Pass so they were fairly close by. They would come to assist me with my day to day duties, cooking for me and taking me to meetings. Good reliable people, there to help and keep me company.

This is where my true friends really came to light, after a few years of feeling betrayed and abandoned. Now, at a time when I needed people the most and after becoming reclusive, the true ones were still there to pick me up where I needed. I found there were more than I thought.

I had been elected to the entertainment chair in my town's recovery group. I was in charge of the sober dances and other events. I was only able to throw one party before succumbing to my disease.

The weekend before Halloween I threw a Halloween party for the recovery group. While at this party, things started going really sideways. During the party I had overflowed my diaper, soiling myself badly. I was covered in fecal matter. Mortified, I went to talk to one of my friends, Mickey, requesting her assistance before others noticed. She took me in the bathroom and helped me clean myself up, after that I was begging to leave. Immediately, they took me home and put me to bed.

On Halloween I was feeling heartsick because one of my favorite things to do is hand out candy to all the trick-or-treaters and their adorable costumes. I couldn't make it to the door because my legs were so bad and I had a ton of candy to give away. I called Jim and Yvette who were close friends from Calgary and happened to live close by. I asked them to come over, close my curtains and shut off all the lights. After they left I sat on the couch and cried myself to sleep.

On November 1st I wanted to go to a meeting, so I phoned a friend and her and her husband picked me up. I had a very hard time walking, I was using my walker but even that was trying. They put me in their car and took me to the meeting. At the meeting they ended up making a judgement call by how bad my disease was and how sick I looked. They would not take me home until I visited a hospital first. I reluctantly agreed, knowing I had no other choice. They weren't going to take me home and I couldn't walk, there weren't any other options. I had no idea that this particular hospital visit would turn into a six month stay.

The Crowsnest Pass Hospital had put me under observation for a day not knowing what to do with me. After a week I was transferred to Calgary Foothills Hospital by ambulance.

Within the first couple of weeks they started me on a treatment called [11]Plasmapheresis which is when blood is taken out of the body through a needle or catheter. The Plasma is removed from the blood

---

[11]    Plasmapheresis is the removal, treatment, and return of (components of) blood plasma from blood circulation. It is thus an extracorporeal therapy (a medical procedure performed outside the body). The method is also used during plasma donation: blood is removed from the body, blood cells and plasma are separated, the blood cells are returned while the plasma is collected and frozen to preserve it for eventual use in the manufacture of a variety of medications. Source: http://en.wikipedia.org/wiki/Plasmapheresis

by a cell separator. When the plasma is separated, the blood cells are returned to the body. The plasma which contains the antibodies is treated and after it is returned to the patient. This required a main line from my throat to my heart. The line would hook me up to an apheresis machine which would take my blood and separate the cells, removing the plasma and replacing it with [12]albumin which would recycle my plasma with clean plasma.

By this point I didn't really know how to feel, I trusted the doctors to fix me and willingly cooperated in every treatment. I did as I was advised. I could no longer ignore my disease.

I had long blonde hair at the time, down to my hips. Because I couldn't get the mainline wet I encountered some issues when it came to washing my hair. The nurses attempted to use dry shampoo, this turned out to be an awful idea. I discovered that I was allergic to the components of the dry shampoo and my eyes swelled shut. I had large hives and my hair was falling out. I had such an awful panic attack it was the first time in my life I had to take any sort of anxiety medication. The reaction was so awful they stopped my treatment for the day.

The treatment worked well for me for the ten days I received it, also for a week and a half after. For someone with typical multiple sclero-

---

12    Albumin is a protein made by the liver. A serum albumin test measures the amount of this protein in the clear liquid portion of the blood. Source: http://www.nlm.nih.gov/medlineplus/ency/article/003480.htm

sis, this treatment could put them into remission for years. However, for me, it only lasted for a week and a half.

After the ten days of treatment and a week of physio they transferred me to the neuro-rehabilitation ward of the hospital, I was elated. I had regained so much of what I had lost and I was giddy about it. I had full functioning legs and my strength was returning.

During my hospital stay, the worse my condition got, the less Craig showed. It was too difficult for him to watch me failing worse. He would visit two or three times a week for twenty minutes so he could wash my laundry for me.

My dear Ralph visited every single day. He would spend two hours taking the bus just so he could spend one hour with me before commuting two more hours home. He always brought goodies with him too.

My parents were frightened and consumed with grief, they felt completely helpless. Another friend of mine named George visited often too, I called him my orange juice dealer. Between Ralph and George, my addictions to fruit and orange juice were well satisfied.

December 2009 was a very sad month for me, I had no choice but to face my disease and there was no more hiding from it. My first inclination that something was terribly wrong was the team of doctors entering my room every day during my stay in the hospital.

At Christmas I was given a pass to stay with my parents, which was wonderful news. I was still having a lot of difficulty with everything beneath my skin. I had regained minimal strength and was already starting to slide back downhill, the treatment was wearing off.

The evening of Christmas Eve my father gifted me a beautiful blanket. It was bright yellow, so cozy, soft and slippery. I adored it.

My parents were helping me into bed that night when I slid off that slippery blanket. I was temporarily paralyzed from the waist down upon hitting the floor. We had to phone my nephew, Michael, who had left earlier after dinner to come put me back in bed. I was horrified, but God bless Michael's soul. He was used to taking care of my family and he lightheartedly lifted me back into bed.

In the evening on Christmas Day I was in the bathroom with my mother. She was assisting me with an enema that I was required to do every 8 hours. I had regained a little bit of strength back from resting all day and I was hunched over the edge of the tub. I should have known better, but my legs gave out and I went crashing to the floor. My legs were completely paralyzed from the moment I hit the floor.

So there I lay, in between the toilet, my mom's wheelchair and the bathtub, completely paralyzed from the waist down with no pants on. My mother hollered for help and everyone raced over to us. The enema was still taking its effect so Teena came in with a dustpan to catch the poop. She shoved it under my ass because the enema was still partially in. My father was on the phone with 911 when they realized I couldn't get up. I was covered in a blanket when the paramedics arrived a half hour later. They loaded me onto a stretcher and brought me to a hospital so they could complete the enema.

As I was leaving the house Teena said, "I can't take this anymore. I can't take care of anyone else anymore."

My heart was broken. I was so mortified and completely distraught as to why these humiliations were so consistent, why was I sliding backwards so quickly? And so soon after I felt liberated that my treatment had worked. I tear up now thinking about it, because even to this day, I still experience many of the same feelings.

My dad picked me up from the Lacombe Hospital and brought me back home. I had the option to be transferred back to the Foothills Hospital in Calgary, but I wanted to go home. It was Christmas after all.

The next day was Boxing Day and also Teena's birthday. She left first thing that morning and didn't come back. Everyone was hurt, especially me. I didn't understand then, but I certainly do now, why she behaved the way she did. She was sick of being around the sick.

I was returned to the Foothills Hospital after my 'vacation'. The doctors were unimpressed with my health and went back to the drawing board, making arrangements to take me out of rehab and switch my meds.

The first week of January in 2010 the doctors had a conference call with my parents. I sat in a conference room with all of my doctors, my parents listening on a speaker. Dr. McGowan, who was the head of the neurological rehab at the Foothills Hospital, was among the doctors. They were discussing what to do with me and what type of MS I had. They thought I had moved from relapsing-remitting MS to secondary progressive MS. They were trying to make sense of my symptoms. I had to listen to my mother and father weep over the speaker in the center of the table. I don't think there is any worse pain for a parent than knowing that your child is seriously ill, with no conclusive diagnosis.

Dr. Pearson, my neurologist in Calgary, came into my room after a few hours and kneeled on the floor to be at eye level with me. She took my hand, explaining that after the meeting with Dr. McGowan, staff and my parents, the decision was made to start me on chemotherapy with a drug called Cyclophosphamide.

"This is all we have left to offer. I can promise you a year, but this is all I can promise. What happens after will depend on your body." She said.

They had already tried the 10 days of plasmapheresis which wasn't effective for me for more than two weeks. The last option on the table was the Cyclophosphamide, and all we could do is pray that it worked for as long as we were hoping.

They knew at this point I was getting close to my demise.

It wasn't easy news to swallow. Craig had retreated before my health had gotten this bad and I knew in my heart he would only get worse. His visits were seldom and I would cry myself to sleep. I didn't understand what I had done wrong. Now I understand it had nothing to do with me, but at the time it broke my heart and made me feel unworthy.

I had my first dose of chemotherapy on January 7, 2010 and within a couple of days they transferred me back to the Crowsnest Pass hospital to be closer to home.

I was hoping that being shipped back to the Crowsnest Pass would encourage Craig to come around more, and possibly see that things were slowly coming around. Slowly is a variant word for me. The treatment was working quicker than I expected, but for him, sick was sick. The progress was nonexistent and he was unhappy, sad and lonely. I'm sure the range of emotions he felt were much more complex but he never confessed anything more to me.

My first two doses of chemo were two weeks apart. I had my second dose on January 22, 2010. I was taken by ambulance to the Lethbridge Hospital for my second dose of chemo and that is where I received my ongoing doses for the next year and a bit. When there was no change after my second dose of chemo, I was feeling pretty sad, let down and afraid. It was one more treatment that wasn't working and I didn't know what to do or where to turn.

On top of everything my bladder was not emptying properly and I also suffered from bladder spasms. They started giving me Botox for my bladder. They spent an appalling fifteen hundred dollars covered by Alberta Health Care just to transport me to a consultation with a urologist back in Calgary. The office was not in the hospital, but in a professional building where they had to carry me on a stretcher up to the examination room. The door of the room would not even close because the stretcher was too long. Absolutely ridiculous. The Botox treatment caused frequent UTI's. My bladder hated me and despised the treatments more.

My third dose of chemo was on February 22, 2010. Between these three doses things were slowly starting to change, I do mean slowly, snail pace slow.

It was somewhere between my second and third dose that my progress slowed to a glacial pace.

I was able to stand in the bars at physio and I knew standing was a start because I hadn't been able to in months. This was exponential progress.

After my third dose things were starting to progress at a faster pace.

I went to physio on a Wednesday feeling excited. I could feel something different within my body and I hoped it would be incredible.

To pull myself up and stand between those bars usually took at least 4 to 5 tries. It took as much effort as I've ever put forth in my entire life just to stand. No aspect of this was easy and I do not in any way, shape or form try to mislead you of the difficulty.

I stood up between the bars and I looked at Calvin, my physiotherapist, and said, "I have a question. Do you think I could possibly try to lift my foot?"

"Of course!" there was shock resonating on his face.

I was excited in a way I hadn't been excited in months. I lifted my foot an eighth of an inch off the floor. Calvin is an excellent physiotherapist and he could see my muscle contract. I may not actually have lifted my foot off the floor but he could see the muscle contract and with that movement he knew this was a good sign. I was overjoyed.

I looked at him excitedly with a grin, "can I try my other leg?"

He nodded, he was as excited as I was.

I lifted my other leg about the same as the first one. I'm neither doctor nor physiotherapist, but I could tell in that moment, being able to lift both feet it wouldn't be long before I could take a step.

The very next day Calvin came and put me in my chair. We went to physio and I repeated the same miracle of miniscule foot movement.

While standing between the bars I was looked to Calvin and I said, "I want to try something different today"

He just smiled.

"Is it possible for me to try to move my leg to the side?"

I was trying to move my foot to the side to see if my hip would move. With this movement I achieved around the same amount as with my feet the day prior. Calvin noticed the muscle contraction again. With that movement, in my heart of hearts, I knew if I could lift my foot move my hip to the side, even just that tiny bit, I would walk again. The barriers had been broken and now all needed was patience.

Calvin took me back to my room and I went to bed exhausted,

resting for the remainder of the day.

Friday morning Calvin came to fetch me and I was beside myself with excitement.

"I have a surprise for you," he said playfully.

I begged him to reveal the secret but he seemed to enjoy making me wait until we got to the therapy room. As we entered, there was an enormous rehabilitation walker parked in the middle of the room. I couldn't wait to use it.

Once I was strapped in and could not fall, I walked an astonishing 30 feet while everyone watched in awe, mouths agape.

I was moving forward much faster than my body could handle and it really took effect over the weekend. I was incredibly sore and all I wanted was to get up and walk more.

I was in so much pain Saturday evening that the nurses wrapped my legs in hot IV bags to settle my excruciating spasms to their best ability. I spent the entire weekend in pain, recovering.

Monday I walked 200 feet, I could not be stopped.

Each day I walked more and more, increasing the distance while Calvin crawled on the floor measuring my steps.

When I reached 450 feet Calvin said, "I'm not crawling on the floor for you anymore."

I had progressed so well with the rehab walker that Calvin gave me a smaller walker with no wheels to work on my balance. I wasn't very happy about this. It was so difficult, I was immediately enraged.

I required two nurses to assist me while I picked the walker up with every step. I was not even close to attaining the distances I had with the other walker.

My hospital bed faced a window which looked out to the highway. Craig was working at the ski shop in Calgary, an hour away from home. I would literally see him drive by without stopping. I would call him and ask him if he was finally coming in to visit and he would brush me off saying he was tired or busy. His visits decreased to once a week, if that, and the only reason why he continued to show up was to do my laundry. Even this was becoming problematic.

I knew I was getting better, I could feel it and if he were around to see the progress perhaps he would feel differently. If only he was willing to share the experience of crossing these enormous milestones with me. He refused to even attempt to see my development, perhaps because he lacked coping skills and maybe he was just flat out selfish. Whatever the reason was, he broke my heart more every day.

My parents tried to visit as much as possible but because of the five hour travel time, and the lack of funds, it was beyond their control. It never stopped them from putting forward their best effort though.

I was basically alone in the Pass. I had moved miles away from my family because I couldn't afford a home in the city, and with a man who now seemed to completely stop caring for me. My denial of my disease blindsided me from thinking too far ahead into the future. I wouldn't have moved so far away if I knew I could get this sick. I was a trucker, I could reside anywhere. I was fortunate to have met some beautiful people that did spare me from complete isolation. They visited and introduced me to new lifelong friends.

A couple of weeks into my physiotherapy with the Godforsaken walker, I was able to use it with the assistance of just one nurse.

I fell down a couple of times because of balance issues and then I would be back to two nurses for a couple more days, then back to one, this cycle repeated a few times.

Soon my progress surged past the two wheel walker to a four wheel walker and I was cruising.

I was in the very early days of strengthening when I met Kyle for the first time. Craig had been stepping further away from me which made people from the recovery program step up.

On a day pass, my friend Barry picked me up from the hospital and drove me to a meeting. Barry's car was small and low to the ground, because of this we had some issues getting me out of the vehicle and into my wheelchair. Kyle, who is acquainted with Barry, came over to offer his assistance and it was greatly appreciated. I weighed over 200 pounds at this point. Over the next couple of months he would become one of the many people who would transport me to and from meetings.

On Good Friday I acquired a day pass from the hospital to paint Easter eggs with some friends and their children. I started to feel unwell and decided I would lie down for a while. When I awoke, I was sweating profusely. I tried to get up from the couch but my legs weren't working, this upset me greatly.

I was burning up with a fever of 105 degrees and my friends raced me back to the hospital. This was three days from my release date. I hallucinated for two of them, losing mobility in my legs. Later on I would find out that this incident was possibly my transition from secondary progressive MS into Marburg's Variant MS. When the fever broke I was beyond perplexed, wondering how on earth and why I was set back so quickly. All of the work and determination, the sheer exhaustion had seemingly been for nothing. What else could I do but sit and cry?

The hospital kept me under observation for another week and that was also the week I made the decision to end my relationship with Craig. My heart was past broken with Craig and now I was just mad. I was done with him.

The next time he came to visit I said completely enraged, "either you pick up those big girl panties or you can get out of my house and make sure you're gone by the time I get home."

As quickly as I had failed, I found my strength again and was able to be released.

When I arrived home, Craig had clearly made his decision, he was gone.

The energy was cold within the house. All of my girlfriends met me there, they brought food and were helping unpack while celebrating this joyous time of being released and finally home. I was looking for my things I had left behind, all those months ago, and I couldn't find anything. I couldn't find my toiletries or personal products. Anything that reminded Craig of me had been put into a box and stuffed into a corner on the top shelf of a closet. When I found it, the feeling that overcame me was one I had never felt before. It was like walking into my house after my own funeral. It felt like I had died and my stuff had been packed away, no longer relevant. I understand his motives now, it was because he couldn't cope, but it didn't make the pain any less.

I was embarking on a new journey with clarity of my health and the trials I would be facing, and I was doing it alone.

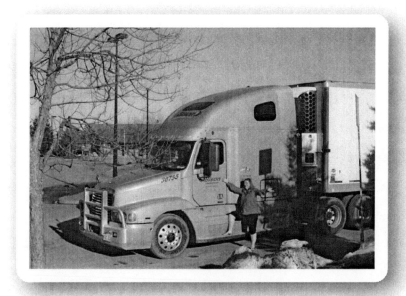

*Me with my Bison truck*

# Sick and Sicker

IN APRIL OF 2010 I WAS HAPPY TO BE HOME AND WORKING ON regaining my independence. Craig was gone and I was happy, but my financial situation still weighed heavy on my nerves. I was aware of the solitude now. Even though Craig didn't offer much support while he was around, at least he was around.

I knew my short-term disability would be running out in June which meant I would have no income whatsoever. If I didn't do something I would lose everything I had worked so hard for. It felt like every time I took one step forward, I'd be dragged three steps back.

I had two spare rooms in my house and decided to rent out one to make the mortgage payments a little cheaper. I rented the room for a low amount to a man that was a friend of a girlfriend of mine. It was all well and good until he ripped me off. He stole many things from me including a $2000 camera. Only three months later he walked out on me without paying his rent.

I was growing tired of making bad decisions.

It seemed everyone who came near me was trying to use me. Terrible people in the world saw my blatant vulnerabilities, I was easy prey.

There were exceptions though, if you give it time, life will attempt to balance itself out. Among the stresses there were many great things still occurring.

I went to physiotherapy every day at the hospital. The few friends I had would drive me to my appointments and I was very grateful for them. They loved me, held me up and did all the things I wasn't able too. They fed, cleaned and coached my spirit, nurturing me with unconditional support. Some were kind people from the church, many were from the program. They all pulled together to take care of me and transport me to my many appointments all over hells half acre.

I knew I had to get back to work by June because my house and basic needs depended on it.

I pushed my body to the limits, striving to recover as quickly as possible. I wrangled up what few funds I had coming in and it turned out there were perks to being so ill. The social worker at the Foothills Hospital was able expedite my application for my [13]CPP Disability Benefits during my 6 month stay. It went through quickly and I was approved instantly. The extra income made it so that I was able to buy myself a used Chevy Trail Blazer. Once this was all in the works,

---

13    Canada Pension Plan

I hired a personal trainer at a gym and was gaining strength back by the day.

I decided to lease the room again to a man who was working on the mines. He was a family man from Calgary that only stayed for the 4 days he was on shift and then he would travel home for his 4 days off. This was a great arrangement. I had a little bit of extra money to feed myself and it felt good not having to rely quite so much on my friends.

I kept in touch with my work and they were starting to set up back to work protocols. This included a list of doctors I needed to see and road tests to do. It was strenuous, but I did it all.

I was literally between a rock and a mountain, to say a rock and a hard place would be an understatement.

I was at the gym five days a week, Evelyn, my personal trainer, was working with me three of those days. I knew the only way to keep going was not to slow down.

My mom often used the 'bull in the china shop' analogy with me; 'go hard or go home' was another regular statement. The theory that there is a thin line between stubborn and stupid is correct when it comes to me. I walked on that line often. I can say I've gotten better since, but I still have my moments.

I used to tell people with conviction, "I'm not stubborn, I'm determined!" just because it sounded better.

All of these analogies paired with my motivating strength and determination had me back behind the seat of my truck by June of 2010.

I was no longer allowed to cross the border because of the risks and the medical expenses should I need hospital care in the US. Another reason was that I was still getting Cyclophosphamide infusions once a month.

The doctors needed to put a PICC line in my arm, which would make it easier for my chemo treatments, this way they could just plug into me. I didn't have time for this though, I was going back to work and the risk for infection would be too high. All medical staff and I got together and decided to put a port (catheter) into my chest that was completely under the skin, this lessened the risk of infection.

In June 2010 I was working in the city. I was driving in on Monday and renting a room at a girlfriends place. The tables had turned. I was leaving my home 5 days a week spending five hundred bucks a month on top of all my other expenses. I was medically only allowed to work a maximum of ten hours each day which is why I had to stay in the city. Coleman is a 2 hour drive from the city and it would have been too much for me to commute daily.

I knew if I could get 24 months in with my work I could qualify for long term disability. Working within the city only lasted six weeks before I was back on short term disability.

The third week of July 2010, my recovery group was having an annual campout. I was home early on a Friday from work and I had gone shopping for ingredients to make a Greek salad for the potluck. While at the grocery store, I slipped and fell under my cart. The stores cooler had been leaking water all over the floor.

A woman who was working watched my fall and came rushing over, "Are you alright?"

"Yes, I'm fine" I said as she helped me up.

She was insistent that I fill out the forms the store had for accidents. I usually wouldn't have done such a thing, but she was persistent. I was lucky she was too; later on I received a settlement for $6000.

It was Saturday and I was at the campout feeling quite ill, apparently I didn't look too hot either. My body was completely swollen. Everyone was buzzing around as I sat with my feet up. My phone rang and it was work asking if I could come in on Sunday morning.

"I can't see why not." I said.

Everyone around me shook their heads and walked away. Remember the stubborn and stupid line?

Here we go.

I drove myself home, convinced if I rested until morning that I'd wake up fine. I did rest and at 5 am I was up with my lunch made and out the door. I arrived at the yard feeling tired, but not too bad. I went inside and found my plans for the day, grabbed the keys for the truck I was driving, hooked up my trailer, did my vehicle inspection and off I went.

I dropped my trailer in the dock, uncoupled and went on the search for empty trailers in the yard to take back with me. By this point I was beginning to comprehend that maybe I shouldn't have come to work.

The empty trailer I needed to take back was behind another trailer. This meant I would have to hook the first one, drop it out of the way and then hook mine and also drop it out of the way. Just thinking about doing all of this made me exhausted. This would require at least ten trips up and down, in and out of my truck. This estimate was only if everything went smoothly, which wasn't common.

I sat with my forehead on the wheel and began to cry, I was so tired and I was so done. I can't explain the amount of fatigue that plagues me while I'm in that sort of shape. I did manage to get it all done, but there was a big price to pay.

I called into dispatch when it was taking longer than it should have. Something like this should have taken an hour at best. I was going on three.

After finally hooking to the right trailer I headed to the yard.

There was road construction in the city on Glenmore trail and pylons were set up between the lanes. I didn't have double vision looking forward, but when I looked in the mirror I was not able to tell which pylons were the correct ones. I called dispatch to let them know I was almost there.

I shouldn't have continued because it wasn't safe in anyway. Since the double vision only affected me while looking in the mirrors I knew I could make the rest of the trip without using them. When I arrived it took me an hour to back in the trailer because I had to use my mirrors.

An old friend of mine, Stephen, whom I used as my emergency contact, came to pick me up. When he arrived I stood and my bladder released. Because of my sensory issues I had no idea that I had even urinated, I couldn't feel it at all. Once the urine reached my feet, soaking my socks, I knew exactly what happened. I asked Stephen to bring me a change of clothes.

Too embarrassed to go in the shop, I changed in a portable toilet. This was a very difficult task to perform in a confined space while weak.

Stephen wanted to take me to a hospital but I stubbornly refused, or should I say I was determined not to go. He took me to his house so he could keep an eye on me and by the time I was on his couch my legs had lost mobility. Stephen's wife, Dana, came home and took one look at me and I knew I was going to the hospital. My determination was no match for hers.

I know I was very ill because I can't recall if they drove me or if I was transported by ambulance, either way, I ended up back in the hospital.

I was admitted to the Rockyview Hospital in Calgary and terrified that this would be another extended stay.

During my stay I met a young man named Brad who had just been diagnosed with MS. He was barely an adult when he received his diagnosis; it broke my heart to see such youth being plagued by this damned disease. He became my friend for the duration of my three week stay and a lifelong friend thereafter. We hung out often, taking our wheelchairs out together and cruising along the lake pathways around the hospital together.

Speaking of great companions, just like clockwork, Ralph would visit me every day.

I only learned recently the reason I was constantly hospitalized and paralyzed.

I used to believe that if I had a fall I would get a UTI and end up temporarily paralyzed. My [14]OT therapist explained that what actually happens is I get a UTI which affects my muscles causing me to have a fall, and then I end up temporarily paralyzed. This makes perfect sense when you think about it, my bladder is my nemesis.

I was placed on short term disability, I went home to the Pass and that's where I stayed until September 2010. By this time I knew the drill, I had to build my strength again before I could return to work. I persisted to achieve this again, working diligent to recover.

While on my short term disability I had a different man move into the room. I won't mention his name because I have nothing nice to say about him. What I will say is that when I went back to work in September I trusted him with my home. I was focused on getting the 24 months in at work and I was barely ever home. I assumed he was sticking to our arrangement as he had been before, paying the bills

---

14     OT: Occupational Therapist

while I paid my mortgage.

I was talking to Kyle regularly, flirting innocently. We spoke on the phone often and I had some inhibitions about our age difference, but continued to befriend him.

The positive effects of chemo started diminishing during October and November, not quite the year I had hoped for. My legs were becoming problematic again and the fatigue was almost unbearable. I pushed on.

I went through thirteen trucks within three months and it was stressful having to transfer all of my belongings from truck to truck each time. I should have read into this as a warning but I was determined.

Everything was beginning to crumble around me. Problems were starting to overlap and I felt as if I were buried in them.

I confided in Kyle often and each time I went to the MS clinic I would relay the jargon of information I received. I didn't know it at the time, but he would google everything I said. He was learning more about me and my disease than I even tried to comprehend at this point. I was still in denial, living day to day, following the doctors orders.

I was growing quite fond of him and asked him to go on a date with me when we had an opportune time.

December 2010 was a hard month on me, I had been given two different trucks and both had exhaust leaks. The first one broke down on me in Grande Prairie; my work brought me another truck and placed the broken one in the shop.

I made it to my parents with the second truck in time for Christmas. I parked it outside their home. There was no doubt in my mind that this Christmas was better than the last, with one exception. My truck wouldn't start again. I had a load to deliver to Cranbrook, BC and ended up waiting for a tow truck on Christmas day. This was a pricey pain in my ass.

Kyle and I finally had our first date on New Year's Eve.

Kyle had wanted to show me the observatory he had built in his backyard for our first date. We were unable to do this because my legs were weak and I couldn't climb the stairs that lead to the observatory. Instead we went to a potluck gathering at a mutual friend's house and it was a lovely evening. It may not have been a formal date but it was perfect for him and I.

I spent the night with him, cuddling in the dark.

He brushed his hand across my face and he could feel me smile and that's when he said, "so long as you can do that (smile) we'll be alright."

It was a blissful evening. I cried my first happy tears in a long while. I was completely and irrevocably in love with him.

I went to Grand Prairie for the New Year, January 2011, and my truck faltered again. Now I had two trucks, in the same city, in two different shops.

I was beyond exhausted, annoyed and just plain infuriated with my luck.

While in my hotel room I felt incredibly ill. Walking from my room to the restaurant took everything I had. If I had been wise, I would have went to the hospital and been put on workers compensation for the remainder of my life.

I was suffering from carbon monoxide poisoning, but I thought the symptoms were just more ailments from my disease. The weather was horrible, my nerves were shot from stress and my disease was reacting.

When I look back now I can see the constant signals, blatantly slapping me across the face screaming, "Fiona! You've had enough!!"

I was stuck in my hotel for two weeks. One of the trucks was finally repaired and I picked it up only to find that the exhaust was still leaking. Being wiser, I didn't take it. I called the company and they set up a time to bring me a brand new Volvo semi, which would be mine for an extended time to follow. This was uplifting news.

The man who brought the new truck kindly transferred all of my belongings for me. Excited about the new ride, I thought maybe, just maybe, this would be the time things would start to change.

I drove in a terrible snow storm from Grand Prairie to Vancouver.

While driving through a mountain pass I could feel my body beginning to shut down. Knowing I didn't have much time, I sucked my pride up and called dispatch.

When Linda answered I asked, "Can you please make sure I get a load back to Calgary out of Vancouver?"

"Why?" Linda was concerned.

"I just can't do this anymore," I felt weepy, "I am done, I have nothing left in me."

Not too long after the initial call, dispatch called back and requested that I go to a hospital in Hope, BC. This was only 20 minutes ahead of me, at the bottom of the mountain.

I parked a half a city block down the road from what I thought was the hospital. I climbed out of my truck and pushed myself to walk to the building. When I finally arrived there I broke out in tears. It wasn't the hospital; it was a long term care facility.

The hospital was still a full city block down the road. I continued to walk, weeping as I did so.

By the time I arrived in the hospital driveway I was crawling, my legs had quit just before the entrance and when my hips quit shortly after. I was flat as a pancake on the sidewalk before I could enter. Luckily, hospital staff saw me and came to my aid. They put me on a stretcher and brought me into the emergency ward.

There was absolutely nothing they could do for me. All they could do was give me a bed to rest and hope I regain some of my strength back.

The next day I was able to take a taxi back to my truck, from there I drove to a truck stop and called dispatch again. I waited two days for someone to fly out so they could drive my truck back for me. During those two days I rested in bed and waited. When he finally arrived, he drove us to Vancouver to drop the load I had been carrying and then we headed back to Calgary.

Once back in Calgary, Kyle came to pick me up with the man who was supposed to be paying the bills and maintaining my house. It was the first time I had been home in four months.

When I got out of the truck in front of my house Kyle stopped me from going in. He had been in the house a couple of times and did not want me to see it.

The man who was residing there was using again and he moved in more drug addicts. He had also discontinued paying the bills that were in my name the moment I left.

He completely destroyed my home and made it condemnable while putting me thousands of dollars deeper in debt. What a complete low life. I mentioned earlier that I had received a settlement for $6000 for a slip in a grocery store; well all of that money went to paying the overdue bills. I was grateful I had the extra money to pull myself out of that situation. It definitely could've been used for other priorities.

I was scared I was about to lose everything I had worked for, and angry that my house had been jeopardized again. I was way too sick to dwell in my emotions though, I just wanted to rest.

Kyle ended up taking me to his home and we've been together ever since.

While staying with Kyle, I learned he was extremely anti-social because he's deaf and has an extremely hard time hearing people speak, it frustrates the hell out of him. When I first met him he was hard to read and he seemed detached with his emotions. I would soon learn that this man had a heart of gold.

Kyle had been single for sixteen years, from the time he got sober until me. Upon deciding to date we were both aware my time was limited. Kyle stayed with me because he loved me, but also because he knew he could let me die with dignity. He cares for me better than any long term care or hospice facility I might be placed in.

Kyle had helped his sponsor while she suffered and eventually passed from cancer. He was there for his best friend's son when he passed away from cancer as well. Kyle was well acquainted with terminal illness and he took it upon himself to be there for me as he had for his loved ones.

I love him more for it. I don't think he anticipated he would fall in love with me, fall in love with someone who was dying.

By the time we met I was in no shape for any kind of love making activities. For this reason we have only actually made love once. The act in itself is painful and leaves little sensation. The spasms would be agonizing. We are emotionally, spiritually and intimately connected like no other. The love we share, most people could not even imagine.

When people ask us how long we've been together he always responds, "twenty-five years." We've only been together for four years at present but you will soon read why this is his response.

My MS symptoms were becoming severe. I was surprised because I didn't think it could get much worse than what I had already endured.

It seemed like every time I said, "It can't get any worse than this" I would have to retract my statement immediately.

I was experiencing [15]'MS hugs', which is a far cry from the warm and inviting embrace the name may sound like. It feels like a constriction around my rib cage, painful spasms while it clenches my diaphragm. With each breath it worsens as I fight for oxygen. I was experiencing them sporadically and they utterly terrified me.

Its other more appropriate nickname is 'the squeeze of death'. Many times its cause is neuropathic but when it's actually activating the intercostal muscles within the ribcage is when it becomes deadly. I was also having 'banding' on areas all over my body at different times. It basically feels like a girdle tightening around whatever part it chooses to hold on to on any given day.

Every symptom that inhabited my body was progressively getting worse. I flailed through to March 2011. My health was spiraling rapidly downhill at a pace I could hardly conceive.

---

15    MS Hug: MS hug is a collection of symptoms caused by spasms in the intercostal muscles. These muscles are located in between your ribs. The muscles serve the dual purpose of holding your ribs in place and helping you move with flexibility and ease. The involuntary muscle spasms Symptoms can last for anywhere from a few seconds to hours at a time. Source: http://www.healthline.com/health/multiple-sclerosis/ms-hug#WhatIsMS1

The most prominent memories I have of this time is my failing health on April 9th.

I had a friend Vicki and the twins over for dinner the night before and it was a lovely, normal evening. She left and I went to bed. When I awoke I was paralyzed from my breastbone down.

I opened my eyes, realizing that I could not move and I was scared, but I didn't panic. I figured it was just another episode and all I needed was more rest.

Kyle wanted to take me to the hospital but I had no desire to be poked and prodded. I knew I could lie in my bed a lot more comfortably at home.

He reluctantly agreed and spent the next two days transferring me from the bed to the couch. The following Monday he went to work and I called my nurse, Kathy, at the MS clinic.

"I think we have a problem – again," was how I started that conversation.

I explained to her what was happening and she could hear the slight labour in my breathing. She scolded me for not going to the hospital but was sympathetic to my reasoning. She had to find me a bed as all the beds in the Foothills Hospital were occupied.

The next morning she called and asked if I could be at the hospital by 5pm, she had finally found me a bed. I agreed and Kyle came home from work to drive me. Kyle called a friend to assist him in transferring me from the house to the truck. They walled me in with pillows just so I wouldn't topple over.

Even in this terrifying and worrisome time I must say that going to the hospital as a high risk patient has its perks. No line, no cover. When we arrived I was immediately placed in a room with a bed and put under observation. Once again, I was in the hospital for another undisclosed amount of time.

The doctors treated my UTI and by day two they put in a [16]central line for a 2nd try with plasmapherisis. This was accompanied by new prescriptions for excessive amounts of drugs. They started me on an excess of medications. The meds seemed to help me improve but they also produced peculiar side effects. A week into my stay I saw what looked like diamonds and ice crystals in my left eye. There they were floating and every so often they would move and form a crescentic shape. They checked me but I wasn't suffering from a retinal detachment.

By the end of April my mind was snapping. This is when I 'lost my bean', that is what I call losing my mind.

My medical file dictates that the doctors weren't aware my mind was questionable until the 7th of May 2010. I know I was feeling off

---

16     Central Line is a long, thin, flexible tube used to give medicines, fluids, nutrients, or blood products over a long period of time, usually several weeks or more. A catheter is often inserted in the arm or chest through the skin into a large vein. The catheter is threaded through this vein until it reaches a large vein near the heart. It is used to administer long term medicine. Source: http://www.webmd.com/pain-management/tc/central-venous-catheters-topic-overview

at the end of April, possibly even before that. I remember lying in bed, anxiously anticipating the Royal wedding which was airing in the early morning hours. I am thoroughly upset that I have no memory of it.

On April 30th my memory is extremely patchy. Looking back, April 30th is the last day I have any clear memories until the end of May.

I was in bed having my last infusion of Cyclophosphamide in a year and a half.

That day I remember Bill, an old friend from the program, sitting beside me. We were chatting about something meaningless. I know I felt uncomfortable with him there. I remember feeling sad and scared.

On May 1st, still confined to the hospital I began feeling puffy with band like pain across my torso.

May 5th, a doctor and I discussed an action plan that consisted of rehab, followed by me making plans for assisted living with the help of the hospital social worker.

May 7th they started my rehabilitation.

Everything from this point on and for the next month is recounted from my medical file notes. During this time I somehow withdrew into myself and into a 'coma'.

It wasn't the type of coma where all is quiet and dismal while my loved ones wait for a response. Physically I was very much there, animated and seemingly stark raving mad.

The same day they removed the central line from my neck I was suffering from very distractible bouts of head shakes.

A week prior to the onset of my vexatious head shakes and prover-bial "loss of my bean" I noticed that my mood was most certainly suf-fering. I felt depressive and tearful, understandable to the situation of course, but it got to the point where it was labelled in my chart as "altered mentality". A couple days passed and around this time they stopped most of my medications. The confusion began to engulf my mind. I had hallucinations, seeing animals including cats and even children.

I was responsive but perplexing staff and visitors with tangential and disjointed speech and being inappropriate with my facial expres-sions. I would sneer and smile maniacally for no apparent reason and at inappropriate times.

The next day proved to be worse than the last, it was noted in my file that my behaviour had become outright bizarre and I was cer-tainly not myself. Unresponsive to questions, uncooperative with ex-aminations and my speech was perseverative.

During my loss of lucidity I regained function of my legs, so much that I was able to walk again. May 9th it seemed I had, physically re-covered miraculously, able to walk again. Yet the more I excelled with my physical strength, the worse my mental status became.

I have vague snippets of memories during a particular episode of regaining my mobility. I got out of bed, slowly and gingerly I headed across the hall to the nurse's desk. I think this all happened in the middle of the night, but I can't be too sure. Originally, I had thought that this was the evening my mind went on vacation. What I do remember from that short walk to the nurse's desk is that it was agonizingly painful, of course it was, I had barely wiggled a toe in a month. There I was, after being a quadriplegic for 3 weeks, getting up out of bed and walking on my own. When I arrived at the corner of the nurse's station they looked at me and there was a collective gasp. Down I went like a wet noodle. After this I retained my mobility but, I could no longer follow commands or retain information.

May 10th I was no longer able to interact in a meaningful way with nursing staff or loved ones. I was talking to ghosts in my room, to friends who were not present. There were moments where I could not even recognize the friends or familiar nursing staff who entered my room.

I can't imagine how Kyle felt watching me confused and uncooperative, with no signs of lucidity. I even teased him by having a reasonable day, having meaningful conversations with him for up to an hour at a time. This was the calm before the storm. That evening I grew agitated and delirious.

While reading the notes from my chart I am horrified, it's like the doctors depict my behaviour like I was the possessed little girl from the movie The Exorcist.

My eyes rapidly fluttered, deviating to the left. I repetitively stroked my 'umbilical' region and withdrew from touch by bicycle kicking with both legs.

The doctors were so taken aback with my bizarre behaviour they contemplated on whether I was suffering from delirium or functional behaviour. They stopped my visitations to see if I was embellishing my actions as a display for attention.

They were likely disappointed a few days later, when they discovered me rolling around in bed, right arm in the air while my left scratched my chest. I did all this just before going rigid with my eyes rolling into the back of my head.

Some nights I climbed out of bed and banged my head against the wall. There were times when I would just lay on the floor, attempting to hide from evil nurses who were out to get me. There was a male nurse who wasn't very nice to me. Later I asked Kyle if this man was real or a figment of my imagination. Kyle informed me the nurse was very real and quite hard on me.

I punched Bill in the face and scratched his hand while screaming, "Get out of my yard!"

Even though I had mentally checked out for a good portion of that time, there are slivers of memory I can recall. During all of them I know I was very frightened.

By the sound of the person I became, it was others that should have been, and were probably afraid. Even now, nobody is willing to share their experience of the animal I became after my bean slipped away.

One of my friends brought me in a little ghetto blaster so I could listen to music. This was a kind gesture because I love music and find it soothing. Had I known that I would start to hear voices talking to me through the radio, I may have rejected the whole device. The voices transmitting through the radio were not demonic, nor did they tell me to hurt myself or others. Instead, it seemed to protect me from that mean male nurse. It would warn me when he was coming to my room and that's when I would lay on the floor.

Eventually I made a formal request for the radio under my bed to be shut off.

I believed one of my nurses was a walking atomic weapon and could see nuclear explosions just outside my window.

One day my doctor tried to conduct an interview with me to gain an assessment on my mental status. I was unable to cooperate. I rocked back and forth in bed, moving my arms in circles. I sat in a sexual position and engaged in repeated pelvic thrusting. It was as if I was possessed by the devil himself. The whole time the doctor conducted his interview I spoke to random people who were not present.

I even thought I was driving, trying to take my seatbelt off before standing. It's no wonder there was an order for [17]Seroquel underneath all of his notes.

I became so aggressive that they had to place me in restraints. I

---

17     Seroquel is an antipsychotic medicine. It works by changing the actions of chemicals in the brain. Source: http://www.drugs.com/seroquel.html

required this on several occasions. The nurse's had me tied down with poesies, funny how deceiving the names of some devices can be. Poesy is a contraption that goes over your body like an octopus. It clamps up under the bed and over your body to the rails. They cinch it up tightly, making it impossible to move. There is a lock in the center of your chest, as far as I can recall, right at the sternum. This allows staff and visitors to go near me without the risk of me biting, kicking or hitting them. I could still spit, and sadly, that's exactly what I did. I was in such an uncontrollable and inconsolable state.

Odd how such things haunt me to this day even though I don't really remember them. Fragments of memory replaying how I tried desperately to get free from my bed that I pulled the oxygen system off the wall.

One evening, Kyle was asleep on a cot on the floor beside my bed. I was still restrained and he woke to me leaning over the side of the bed. I stared at him eyes wide with a menacing smile, strands of drool dripping to the floor.

How he continued to stay with me day in and day out after that terrifying incident I will never be able to comprehend. If this is not the definition of unconditional love, I don't know what is.

In my fragments of memory there was a moment when hospital staff were attempting to give me an MRI. I had no idea what contraption I had been placed inside of and I was fearfully trying to claw my way out. The MRI was unsuccessful. They could not get a clear image. They had no answer to their theory that my mental break was possibly a result from viral encephalitis. After this episode I retreated back to my dream world.

I came to in the 3rd week of May. I saw that my room was void of all the love and good wishes that were there. Before I slipped into the place I don't like to think about, my room had been full of cards, flowers, fruit baskets and pictures. Now they were all gone. Many of them I had destroyed with my own hands before they could be removed. Also nowhere to be found was Kyle, his absence was the first I noticed. I knew he was gone, I could feel it. My room was so cold, nothing to do with the temperature, just barren.

I was always surrounded by love and in this moment I had never felt so alone.

One gift in particular I received was from my friend Trysh's daughter. It was a beautiful picture she painted for me to hang at the foot of my bed. I adored it and in one of my tangents (that I don't remember) I took it off the wall and smashed it to smithereens. There are so many feelings that I hurt and I want to apologize for, but I'm not able to because it wasn't me doing those awful things. The list of people needing apologies was endless, the nurses and doctors, my friends, my parents and Kyle.

While I was on my mental vacation, there was a massive fire in northern Alberta that burned the entire town of Slave Lake. When I heard about it and whenever I hear about it, it feels surreal. I now understand how people feel when they have been lost in a world other than their own. I feel like I understand amnesia in the truest sense of the tragedy. Lost time really is just that, lost time. It still breaks my heart to think of the things I missed, even though I didn't know I had missed them at all.

On May 27th I was admitted to the psychiatric ward of the Foothills Hospital. I wasn't transferred until the 30th and by then my wits had already begun returning to me.

While spending time in the confines of my mind I thought I was dreaming. I had been in dreamland for days - weeks. I had 4 or possibly 5 different dreams running all the time. It was like I was able to jump between them all at my own will.

Something I learned about Schizophrenics while being one is that while in a dream state, I'm able to shift through dreams. To elaborate on this, there are good and bad sides to all dreams, if I get scared or nervous in one I can switch sides in that dream or change dreams all together. It really is quite nifty, the power of the mind. I was completely mad on the outside, but completely in control within.

One of my dreams was of a meeting I went to all the time. I had different feelings about it. My mind and, in many ways my life, is very black and white. This was abundantly clear and identifiable in my dreams. When I was within the black I would go as far as to say I was not a very nice person. While in my crazy state, I felt free to think and speak freely of my feelings whether they were good or bad. Unfortunately, I think the harsher thoughts and actions of my 'dreams' projected through to reality and made me all the more insane.

Another one of my dreams I was a bad princess and my sister was the good princess. How despicably accurate this felt for me.

In this dream I was drinking again and fighting with everyone. I think in reality I was fighting with security guards out front of the hospital.

Yet another dream I was a Danish farmer who wanted only to be in the dirt, yet I was in the hospital. It was not reality but I have not overlooked the irony. I could see Kyle as I looked out my window. He was far out of my reach, down in the field and in the dirt. I couldn't get to him because I was behind the glass, confined to my room. In this dream I was sad most of the time because I couldn't reach Kyle.

I remember my first conscious thought upon exiting dreamland was [18]Hatfield's & McCoy's.

I didn't realize how many mixed feelings I had dwelling inside me. Being locked in my mind showed me many things. I truly believe it has changed me for the better in many ways.

On my first conscious day I woke up and got out of bed. I sensed that somewhere inside I was still very broken, but I was recovering and that had to count for something.

---

18    Hatfields & McCoys is a three-part 2012 television miniseries based on the Hatfield–McCoy feud produced by History channel. Source: http://en.wikipedia.org/wiki/Hatfields_%26_McCoys_(miniseries)

I went into the bathroom to call my mother on my cell phone because I thought the nurses and doctors were taping my conversations from the desk.

I cried for my mother's help. She had to do something because I believed I was going to be locked up for good. As I recall this, I can't imagine how difficult that call must have been for her. How helpless she must have felt listening to me, crying while she had no answers for me.

I asked for my dad and she sent him to save the day. He is, was and will always be my savior. He raced from Tees to Calgary to find out nothing could be done for me.

I watched him as he sat in the hall in his wheelchair, tears streaming down his cheeks as two orderlies walked me away. This was that last time I would see him for an entire year.

They locked me in the psychiatric ward on the 27th of May. I learned quickly that I wasn't allowed off the unit, not even to step in the hall to get some air.

I don't think I had felt a breeze, let alone took a breath of fresh air for quite some time by this point. They took my cell phone and anything I could hang myself with, and this was remarkable to me. These people didn't know me at all. I couldn't even talk to my parents because their number was long distance. I could barely remember any of my friends phone numbers but the few I did spread the word which gave me a few visitors.

Kyle was long distance too, even though that didn't matter now because I believed he was gone. He did come visit me one more time to tell me the doctor thought I was dangerous and probably wouldn't get my sanity back.

He asked, "Are you still hearing voices?"

"Sometimes," I answered honestly. I knew that admitting this would mean he would give up on me.

He stood up and walked away. I felt lost, sad and defeated. Heart sick again, I was devastated. Now I was stuck in the psychiatric ward for an undetermined amount of time, alone.

I had never been around mentally ill people before, and now I was surrounded by them. This was an entirely new setting for me. There were some people in the unit that were just a little off, like me at this point, but then there were some that could have been like me a few weeks prior, only now heavily medicated.

I discovered that the mentally ill can be quite messy. Untidy like I have never seen before. They would open things and spill the contents with no concern for the mess, then walk away. I spent many hours cleaning up after them. I also started to re-label the cupboards that had their labels torn off. This is how I started to figure out I was coming back from the 'bad place'.

I was doing all I could to keep busy and stay away from all of them and with that notion I knew I was back. I spent a lot of time on the treadmill which was another place I could be secluded. In the back of my mind I knew that I was still too close to crazy to trust myself. I was terrified to be sucked back in there, inside of my head, not knowing when or if I would return.

Friday, the 3$^{rd}$ of June, I had a meeting with one of the staff psychologists. He told me that I needed to stay for a couple more weeks because they were going to have a meeting with a group of doctors.

Being completely restricted and confined from venturing outside the unit I panicked. "I need out, I need out!" I said as he tried to calm me, "I am not like these people, can't anyone see this? I do everything away from them to avoid being sucked back into that terrifying place! - Please, PLEASE!" I begged desperately.

Something in all my ranting and pleading made him reconsider his decision. He did some investigating that morning, speaking with my physiotherapist from the main hospital that knew me before my lapse of sanity.

She came to visit me while I was on the treadmill. We talked while I walked and she was amazed by my physical progress.

Saturday I got up and went about my day in the crazy place with the not so well crowd. I was lucky too, I had visitors. My friend George came to see me, also Dave and Gena. Dave and Gena asked if I could get a day pass to attend the MS walk in the morning. I had completely forgotten all about the event and that I had been raising funds for the walk before my mental break.

I looked at them sadly, regretfully knowing that the answer to that question already. After the meeting with the psychologist yesterday, there was no hope, they wouldn't even let me into the hallway outside the unit. Dave and Gena were more optimistic than I at this point.

"Can we go ask? The worst they can say is no."

They had a point and I didn't argue.

We walked over to the charge nurse and I asked, "Do you think there is any chance what-so-ever that I could be given a day pass to go with my friends to the MS walk in the morning?"

"Let me call the doctor," was her response.

I was taken aback. She was actually taking the time to make the call, it put me right back on my heels. I heard her ask and I saw her nod and smile at me. It turned out I was supposed to have been transferred back to my home hospital yesterday.

She relayed the doctor's message that I was to leave the hospital as early as I could in the morning, and to return as late as possible. I would be transferred back to the Crowsnest Pass hospital first thing Monday morning.

My wonderful friends picked me up bright and early the following morning and took me to the walk. We spent all morning at the MS walk. My friend Stephan, who had been one of the few numbers I knew off by heart, came to pick me up at the walk. He had helped me out during much of my psychotic break.

I spent the rest of that Sunday with him and his family. They took me back to the hospital after supper around 8pm.

Monday, June 6<sup>th</sup> at 11 am I was in an ambulance being transferred back to the Crowsnest Pass Hospital.

A couple of years later I would have a dear friend who also has Multiple Sclerosis. My friend had the misfortune of experiencing a mental break as well. Her break aroused so many questions pertaining to what the actual cause of it was. Because it was never clear why. The doctors had speculated several aspects as to why I went stark raving mad but there were never any conclusive findings. How many patients really have to go through this? It was too close to home.

While in discussion with this friend he used a statement that made more sense to me than any before, "We use our last memories to construct our own reality while in that state of mind."

While I was schizophrenic I survived within my dreams. I had no actual memories of reality. It was hard to recollect even the faintest memory from my most 'lucid' day during that month.

Getting back to where I left off, I was lying in a bed after being transferred back to the Crowsnest Pass hospital. It resonated that this would be the last time I would be returned here. I had been told that it was time I go home and get my affairs in order. There was nothing else they could do for me.

I was in my room a few days before I made the decision to call a lawyer and get started on those affairs. This is not a call a woman of 38 takes lightly and I was overwhelmed with grief.

Most are familiar with lawyers and their stereotypes. Mine charged me $75 to travel 2 blocks from her office to my bedside.

She sat with me and asked me question after question pertaining to my final wishes. The questions she asked me, sadly, were quite generic for my situation.

She was just there to do her job and that is exactly how it felt. I was disheartened that this very delicate situation for me could be just another day, another dollar, for her. I was so used to being spoiled by everyone with their attentiveness to my feelings. I found her dismissive attitude and nonchalant demeanour quite disconcerting. How could she be so aloof while I was making preparations to die?

I missed Kyle immensely. When I finally found the courage to call him, I was surprised that he sounded glad to hear from me.

Kyle and his friend Don were coming home from Lethbridge when we spoke. They stopped by to check out how high the spring runoff was flowing over Lumbreck Falls. I remember feeling bitter that he wasn't headed straight to me instead of stopping at the falls.

It felt like I hadn't seen him in months, when in reality it was only a few weeks.

I am grateful he believed me when I said I wasn't crazy any more. He could tell on his own from the way I spoke and the sound of my voice. Knowing why didn't matter much to me. What did matter is that he knew and now he was back in my life once more.

In the 2nd week of June 2010 I was released from the hospital.

Kyle took me back to his place and I found it difficult to call it home again. Because Kyle was under the assumption I wouldn't recover from my crazy spell so he had continued on with his life like I was no longer a part of it.

It wasn't easy for either of us to digest. When I arrived home all of my stuff was packed into boxes, all ready to be taken back to my house. From there he was prepared to walk out of my life completely.

Words cannot explain how grateful and relieved I felt that this was not the series of events that took place. Kyle and I talked, cried and laughed. We were opening up to grow into what we are today. Standing side by side, battling together and fighting for each day. We decided that from this point on, even though I was dying, we were going to enjoy every moment that we had left together.

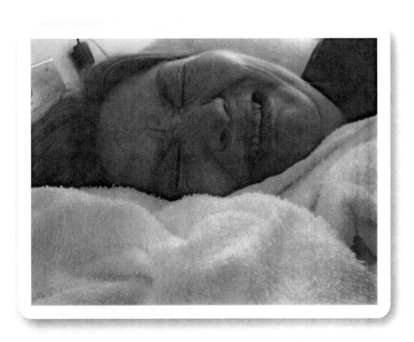

*I don't know who took this picture, but this is the
epitome of my mental break.*

# The Red Light

MY MOTHER HAS A FRIEND NAMED ANNE STEWART. THIS FRIEND-
ship would ultimately add precious time to my life. Anne Stewart was
the head of the MS society in Lethbridge, AB.

In June of 2011, the day after the annual MS walk, I was transferred
back to the Crowsnest Pass hospital. I met Anne for the first time in
my first week there. Up to this point, I had known her by reputation
only. She had just reinstated the Crowsnest Pass MS support group in
January of 2011. It was this group where I had the pleasure of meeting
her. My first meeting with her took place at a time when I had just
been diagnosed with Marburg Variants MS. Revealing this information to Anne would prove to be a miracle in itself.

Upon hearing of Marburg's Variant she said, "I have worked at the
MS society for twenty five years and I have never heard of that term."
At that time I knew as much as she did about it.

Many terms exist for my form of MS including. Marburg's Variant,

Acute Fulminant, Malignant, Tumefactive MS and others. It is an understatement to say that if any of the other terms had been used in this account, this book would not exist.

For a long term, Anne had been following [19]Dr. Freedman, a professor of medicine in the field of neurology at the University of Ottawa in Ontario. He is also a director of the Multiple Sclerosis Research Unit at the Ottawa Hospital. She attended all of his seminars and followed his work closely.

When she went home to Lethbridge she did some research of her own on Marburg's Variant.

She learned that Dr. Freedman would speak about his research at the Consortium for Multiple Sclerosis Centers, CMSC annual conference in Montreal, Quebec. Anne and Lorraine, who is the head of the MS Society in Red Deer, reserved their seats at the lecture. They made the trip from Alberta to Montreal in June of 2011 to attend the talk.

Dr. Freedman gave a fascinating and inciting presentation. He spoke of his completed bone marrow transplant study. They no longer offered the procedure, he said. He said he would not be performing any more transplants. He would however make, he added, an exception for someone with Marburg's Variant.

---

19      Dr.  Freedman  Biography  Source:  http://www.ohri.ca/profile/
msfreedman

Anne's ears must have rang when Dr. Freedman said Marburg's Variant.

Incredulously, this new term had been presented twice within just a few weeks. She was no doubt excited for me. Suddenly before her, this new door had suddenly opened. Fate had knocked and good fortune continued. Later that same day Anne and Lorraine ran into Dr. Freedman at a street corner. They had both stopped for a red light, waiting to cross the street. As they waited, Anne spoke to Dr. Freedman, mentioning myself to him.

Tell her to contact me immediately, he told Anne.

This marked the entry point of the journey I would undertake.

Anne called and excitedly told me, "You need to reach Dr. Freedman's research nurse! There's something that can be done for you. I don't know what will come of it but you need to get a hold of them."

I couldn't help but feel excited by the elation in her voice. Jotting down the information for Marjorie, Dr. Freedman's research nurse, I emailed her immediately. As I waited for her reply, I burned with every emotion: fear, anxiety, excitement, you name it.

After ten days of waiting, I had received no response. My health was depleting rapidly and I knew, I knew I was dying and I took it upon myself to call Marjorie. I could wait no longer. When I called she answered, fortunately.

She cut me off before I could finish introducing myself saying, "I was just about to call you!"

She told me I needed to round up all of my medical files and have them sent to their office in Ottawa.

Over the next week, I spoke with all of my doctors. They sent to Dr. Freedman's office all the necessary paperwork including a referral. While waiting for my paperwork to be sent to Ottawa I had more medical testing to complete. Ottawa needed to know if the inside of my body was strong enough to withstand the transplant. This required an echocardiogram and a whole gamut of lung testing.

A couple of weeks passed. I grew increasingly agitated and impatient. The suspense was killing me. Then Marjorie finally called me back. She and Dr. Freedman had time to go over my information. Later I came to learn just how much work they had to put in, something I didn't realize at the time, to arrange provincial funding for me to go to Ottawa for the procedure.

They setup a date for meet and greet with Dr. Freedman and Marjorie, which would be financed by Kyle.

At the end of July 2011 Kyle and I flew to Ottawa, my emotions, a flurry of erratic hypersensitivity. I did not know what to expect. That a possibility existed I could be saved seemed too good to be true. I'm no fool when it comes to reality, if it looks too good, experience seems to have taught me, it likely is.

Meeting Marjorie and Dr. Freedman for the first time was nerve-racking. Dr. Freedman looked intimidating as he stepped into the room. Looming above me over six feet, he exuded power I could never have imagined any human being possessed.

This man held my life in his hands. I could feel the weight of the situation. I had no guarantee that he would accept me as a patient. Whether I was a suitable candidate for the procedure that would possibly extend my life, only he alone had the power to decide.

He looked me over. "You are lucky you're the sickest of the sick," he said, "or we would not be able to accept you for this transplant."

Many would have been disappointed with that statement, but I was overjoyed and relieved. With that one statement, death was no longer imminent. I now I had a fighting chance, which was all I could ask for.

We discussed the procedure and made arrangements to come back to meet the specialist team, who would perform the procedure. This wouldn't be for another month. Kyle and I flew back home. There I walked as much as my body and the steroids would allow. To have the procedure I had to be able to walk 100 feet. I pushed myself to the absolute limit, determined to make it. In accepting me, they had done their part. Now I had to do mine.

*SEPTEMBER*

My steroids ran out and wore off just before we left for Ottawa at the end of August 2011 for the second meeting with the hematology team. I had also recently been diagnosed with a yeast infection. What terrible timing. My body had again begun its quick deterioration, and again I was temporarily paralyzed, requiring assistance on and off the plane. I was terrified. After coming so close to salvation, I thought, now I would for sure be rejected. Kyle assisted me off the plane. We headed straight for the Rotel which, is a hotel owned by the rotary club and directly across the street from the hospital. They offer discounted rates for out-of-towners who are visiting doctors. Thank God for this.

Sitting in the room of the Rotel, I wept in self-pity but managed to pull myself together in time for the appointment a couple of days later. I met [20]Dr. Atkins, the head of the hematology team that would be doing the procedure and an Associate Professor of Clinical Hematology at the University of Ottawa. He was unhappy that I wasn't walking. Once again, here stood another man with the power over my life in his hands. He made a decision that day that saved me again, by not letting me go home. He knew as well as I did that if I had gone home, I wouldn't have come back. Kyle and I went back to the Rotel to wait for him to set up a treatment for me. For the following eight months, the Rotel would end up being our residence.

My cousin Stacy, who knew I would be staying for an extended period, created a blog for me and taught me how to post to it. The blog

---

20      Dr. Atkins source information: http://www.ohri.ca/profile/hatkins

was to keep friends and family connected as well as to raise some money for the impending costs. While trying to let my unknown followers get to know who I was, I didn't anticipate all of the memories that I would be stirring up. While reminiscing I was facing some self-confrontations and it was rather painful.

On September 4, 2011, Dr. Atkins started me on a potent type of chemotherapy called [21]Mitoxantrone. This form of chemo is so strong it is usually administered once every three months, but he prescribed two doses within six weeks.

The Mitoxantrone was so potent it knocked my immune down low enough that my body was no longer attacking itself. After this I was able to roll to my side and walk behind my chair 150 ft. It was astonishing that, even with the chemo fog that settled over my brain and left me feeling I had little intellect, I was grateful to regain some mobility.

A few days into blogging, I realized that my life, ailments and all, was not very exciting. Sharing news of my profound ability to move with friends and family was great, but to those who didn't have an emotional stake in my progress likely viewed the details on my blog as rather mundane.

Mundane or not, September 7 I took it upon myself to get my feet off of my chair and test my balance. I have instinctual feelings often

---

21    Mitoxantrone, for more information visit: http://chemocare.com/chemotherapy/drug-info/Mitoxantrone.aspx#.VPYcXvnF91Y

of my capabilities. They are like tiny miracles and testing my balance proved to be one. I was improving and that alone was a miracle. Unfortunately, such tiny miracles and good occurred with a sporadic inconsistence. Every time I managed to reach up and grasp firmly onto anything, I would fall back landing flat on my ass.

During such setbacks, it was Kyle I had to rely on. It tormented me to have him assist me –a grown woman with an independent mind - as if I were a child. My torment caused me to sink a state of mixed emotions, pushing me into old selfish habits that made me forget that other people had feelings too. Even now I find this hard to admit.

Early in our stay in Ottawa, Kyle and I developed a routine of every morning going from the Rotel to get coffee at the hospital. To the coffee shop and back to our room was 3 km trek. On weekends, when the hospital coffee shop is closed, it was a 5km roundtrip to the nearest coffee shop. Kyle functions best with set schedules; I despise them. I let him have his way with the schedule though; I need him to thrive, something that I was attempting to do. We walked as much as possible just to escape our confining room.

For practicing my steps, I began to walk in a hallway in the children's hospital that was connected to the Ottawa General Hospital. After one productive day I felt confident like a peacock, and I looked forward to do some more practices. In my cockiness, I foolishly ignored the numbness in my legs, and began to walk, my feathers cocked proudly. I must have looked awfully silly when I crashed to the floor after 3 steps. Commotion ensued. People rushed to my aid. Kyle tried to calm them, reassuring our good Samaritans that I would survive. Bruises, Kyle and I knew, were the least of our problems. I got right back up and went for it again, and I was able to walk 150 feet.

Throughout these daily treks and practice, with the aim of regaining my mobility. I grew anxious that Marjorie, across the street, had forgotten about me. The absence of my friends and family, even early in my stay, started weighing heavily on me.

On September 9, Kyle and I rented a walker. It had brakes that would take effect when you leaned down on the walker, which was good because it lessened the chances I would tip over. To walk my 150 feet, Kyle took me on a 5 km roundtrip to the Walmart and then to the hall. We stopped briefly so that poor Kyle could rest his legs. Then we ventured back out again to test out my walker. I tried out my walker, slowly, across rough pavement and unlevelled bricks. Once again, to some this may seem mundane, but for me it was a great personal achievement.

On September 10 I made it 675 ft. with three five minute rests. I was on a roll and I had no desire to slow down, let alone take a breather. Kyle knows me, including my body, better than I will accept. It frustrates him to no end when I have no desire to listen and then I end up waking up exhausted, and this happened often.

That familiar MS fatigue was hitting me like a ton of bricks on that day, and my lower limbs weren't functioning once again. The extra exertion sent my muscles in spasms and angry knots. I felt frustrated. I'm not sure how Kyle endured my frustrations, but it wasn't the first time and it wouldn't be the last. I had never spent more time with anyone in my entire life than I was with Kyle in Ottawa. I find it remarkable we both lived to tell about it.

Despite everything, Kyle continued to help me out of the room every day and into the walker. I walked as much as my body and Kyle allowed. I even started physiotherapy and found I could still receive new information on learning how to walk again, after I had learned three times already. There were more exercises to add to my regime.

One beautiful day Kyle and I decided to take a stroll through a massive park not too far from the hospital. We ended up getting lost. As a result, Kyle walked over 25 km that day. I need add here that because of having to push me most of the time, Kyle had to endure an awful amount of walking. His resilience is unlike anyone I have ever met.

We went for walks in the morning for our coffee, I attempted walking in the hall of the Children's Hospital and I practiced my stretches and exercises three times a day. One exercise, with which I struggled greatly, required me to sit and stand in a chair. All I needed to do was stand all by myself and then perform a controlled sit. The things we take for granted.

In all I did, Kyle always cheered me on, challenging me to perform more exercises during our walks. We made bets on who could beat who in our trips to the coffee shop, given he had to return my walker to the Rotel first. One time I beat him rolling 1500 ft. on top of 600 ft. I had already completed. My muscles grew angry and ached as I engaged in the competition - but it had no effect on my pride.

On September 16, unable to get my legs out of the shower, I cried the entire day. Kyle gave me extra TLC but as I continued to weep, my emotional state thwarted his efforts to help me. Kyle is my blessing and yet I make him sad when I cry all the time, I wish I could find a way to show him how much he means to me; how amazingly grateful I am to him for the way he had taken this sick little bird under his wing, trying to bring her back to life. God sure puts people where they are needed. He has done that for me, he has put Kyle beside me. Angels come in different forms. In my life they look, smile and laugh just like Kyle.

Because of the frequent UTI's that beset me, an infectious disease specialist was added to the team of doctors that gathered every Monday for a 'Fiona Meeting'. The UTI's became such an issue; fear gripped me that I would be sent home untreated.

As if the UTI's weren't enough, one evening we ended up in the emergency room. my catheter had come out. I remember the look of shock on Kyle's face as he stared at the end of the catheter that was supposed to be inside me. I was grateful I couldn't feel the lower half of my body at that time. Kyle could write an entire novel about his adventures as my caregiver.

Kyle and I decided to take a trip to the Science and Technology museum in Ottawa. I suffered a powerful MS hug afterwards, fatigued beyond words. I noticed a trend with any glorious outings I participated. I always ended up 'paying for' them.

I signed up for acupuncture, hoping it would resolve some issues I had with my sensation. I had noticed numbness around my stomach and fingers.

Much aware that the chemo would result in hair loss, I had Kyle take me for a haircut. We laughed about it. Knowing he would be the next person to give me a trim, Kyle got a kick out of it.

I will forever be grateful for the humour Kyle brings to my days. That I can laugh with him is a blessing next to none. I can't find enough words, nor are there enough words to express how loved and how well I'm taken care of I am. My only sadness comes from how I often say things I regret. The words come out so fast, before I am able to shut my trap, words that hurt Kyle. He does so much for me that the moment those hurtful words escape my mouth, words I cannot take back, I feel utterly lost. I need to learn how to shut up, something that has never been in my make-up.

The team prolonged my treatment for another week. That made me bitchy, and almost intolerable. Kyle, the only one present, was there to share all of my highs and lows. Some of those lows, unfortunately, came with some very harsh blows. My patience was wearing thin. I wanted to be better yesterday!

My body was improving, growing stronger. A time came when I could push on my toes and lift my heels. At one point I succeeded to pull my ankles towards my head while laying down.

My acupuncturist told me the treatments seemed to be accelerating my improvement. I walked 168 ft. uphill and 135 ft. downhill. Going downhill was much more difficult, it requires the use of more muscles to fight gravity.

I found out my mother had been hospitalized for complications with her MS. I felt helpless that I was so far away unable to do anything. I looked like a young Alzheimer's patient, while my mother was in the Lacombe hospital I kept calling the Didsbury hospital. I insisted to the lady answering the phones that my mom was taken there by ambulance the day before. This was lunacy because my folks had left Didsbury 18 years prior.

I never forget how lucky I am because my beloved Kyle always makes sure to spoil me with the little things, like watching sunsets, brisk walks through the park, bird watching and even moving benches to accommodate me in the sun so he can still sit in the shade.

The good and troublesome seemed to take turns in my life. For three days in a row, I was able to walk all three days. Two of those three days I was able to dress myself. By the fourth day, I could not dress myself. Then back to square one I went. This was my life, nothing new.

One day along the walking path, Kyle and I met a nice couple named Joan and Neil. They posted to my blog a nice poem about strength they had written.

"Life is a battle to lose or win.

Are you a fighter or do you give in?

Never acknowledge despair or defeat.

Fight your way forward and never retreat."

This kind of thoughtfulness really helps to renew faith in humanity.

On September 26 Kyle rented a car so we could go see the leaves in Quebec. The weather was wonderful. There wasn't a cloud in the sky. It was such a glorious day that although we did end up getting lost at one point in, it hardly bothered us. I did seven side steps at a rail in Pink Lake and I was in and out of the car over a dozen times that day.

However, the end of the day brought tears. When we returned to our room, the nurse had no new messages waiting for me.

The Rotel we stayed in cost us $350 each week and with Kyle digging deeper into his savings it became imperative that I be admitted. I pushed myself that evening and with the assistance of my walker, I succeeded to walk 66 feet through a rough and soggy gravel lot.

The next day I walked 250 feet after Kyle pushed me through a park, my catheter bag was dragging on the ground for God knows how long. It was at this point that it became absolutely necessary that we pick up new handle covers for my wheelchair, since by now Kyle was pushing me roughly 10 km each day. What a trooper.

Kyle and I knew that my hair would be gone soon. He insisted I wear his toque since it was autumn and the weather would only get colder. I didn't like his toque because it looked just like a long shore man's hat. Grateful to have coverage for it, I purchased some cute hats from a woman who made them specifically for chemo patients. She fit the caps to my head while I still had lots of hair which turned out to be a bad idea. If you are ever, God-forbid, in the market for chemo caps, buy them after your hair is gone. Another thing, buy them in season so you don't freeze or cook in them. I was also able to find other treasures. You know how sickly you are when finding a pill box that's large enough to fit four different slots for each seven days gets you elated.

I desperately tried to make myself better with any resource available. Sure, the doctors could help me, but I understood that I had to work twice as hard. To prove that I deserved the help I was getting, at least this was how I felt because my life depended on it. Within my first month of being in Ottawa I had used up all of my $350 coverage for both acupuncture and physio. The acupuncturist was five miles away from the hospital, and it had meant more walking for Kyle. We didn't have a vehicle. I need to stress that throughout our entire stay in Ottawa, Kyle's feet, back, blood, sweat and tears were my transportation.

As time went by I became restless waiting to find out what was happening. My situations had been kept on the fence, as to whether or not I would be accepted for the transplant. As I waited anxiously, I don't think I could handle being rejected.

I often told my sponsees, "If you don't want the answer, don't ask the question."

After agonising on it, I finally got the nerve to call Marjorie. I asked what was going on.

"Are you back up to your baseline?" Marjorie asked. A baseline is basically the level of 'normalcy' before new harsher symptoms occurred. I had not had a stable baseline for over two years, pushing three.

Unsure how else to answer, I said, "I am able to walk with my walker every day, some days more than others."

She understood and booked me an appointment for the following Thursday for a second dose of Mytox, so I could continue what we were doing. How well the Mytox would work only time would tell.

*OCTOBER*

By October I succeeded to walk 60 feet all by myself without a walker, plus another 150 feet using Kyle and the railing for assistance. I gained weight too, twenty to thirty pounds even as I consumed vast amounts of fruit. Kyle, of course, ventured out every day to bring me more. Because of my weak immune system, I wasn't allowed to touch anyone or anything. This proved to be a difficult process not just for me but for Kyle as well. Keeping a watch on me, he had to constantly remind me and scold me not to touch people. I never realized before how much I did that.

One evening after a walk Kyle and I returned to our room to find a message on the answering machine. In the message, Dr. Adkins nurse said we were booked for 9am the following morning. I assumed things would be changing rapidly.

They didn't.

The treatment took longer than anticipated. By Thanksgiving Kyle and I could feel the pain of isolation. We were far away from our families. With Christmas approaching, the pain would only grow. I had never spent a Christmas away from my family. It broke my heart to think that this would be my first one without them.

On Thanksgiving we spent time walking through central Ottawa. We watched people, admiring the beautiful shades of autumn. We had dinner in the cafeteria, turkey with all the fixings. We talked about what we were grateful for. We had many things. First and foremost we were both grateful for my second chance at life. We were too, grateful for each other. We were also very grateful that we hadn't murdered each other yet. After dinner, I walked 210 feet. Kyle said my walk resembled 'a very drunk girl hanging off a railing with one hand and sometimes two'. Stumbling or not, I was walking. I would be grateful for that, if nothing else. We were quite lucky that Thanksgiving weekend. We experienced record-breaking beautiful weather in Ottawa. Indulging, we spent as much time outside as my body would allow us. I was fortunate that the chemo had been prolonged to go past this weekend. That allowed us to venture out for an entire day. Instead of lying in bed sick from treatment, I was able to enjoy nature at its finest. As beautiful as our treks were I'm sure Kyle was exhausted from having to push me over ten miles in that one day. I told him he should continue to enjoy the sights after I was bed-ridden without the burden of pushing me around, but he disagreed.

Kyle had lived a fairly solitary life before he came to be with me, and now he was thousands of miles away from home, stuck with me almost every second of every day. He had sacrificed his time and money for me and now his sanity, it appeared, would be next. But I cherished his companionship. I loved the feeling as he cuddled next to me before bed so much that I hated waking alone because he could get no sleep due to my snoring. But thank heavens for blessings. Kyle's sense of humor is able to lighten even the dimmest of moods, especially when I descend into consuming moments of aggravating self-pity. I was still struggling with horrible spasms, no doubt from my strenuous efforts. The need for these draining efforts caused me to be very angry, mainly due to frustrations I felt with myself. Most of the time I am aware of the underlying causes of this anger. Only three situations can bring it on; when I'm hurt, scared or I want something I can't have. In my case, I was suffering from all of those situations. My body was physically hurting me. The thought of failure that would surely result in death terrified me. I wanted so desperately, but futile-ly it seemed, to be healthy again.

I felt blessed to have Marjorie assist me with my vast questions. She guided me benevolently through each one. She possessed more patience than I have. Despite my efforts, I didn't have a lot of faith in my own capabilities. I required constant reassurance and consolation.

The ups and downs from trying to regain my strength left me sit-ting in my chair pouting on more than one occasion. I was becom-ing temperamental, a flurry of mixed emotions brewing inside me. I found solace being outdoors where I could be surrounded by the thriving life of nature and people. It was refreshing and I enjoyed taking pictures. I like to capture moments even if they only seem meaningful to me.

In case my treatment overlapped with my birthday, Kyle took me gift shopping. He wanted to make sure I could enjoy myself. With a brand new pair of slippers and socks to keep my frozen feet warm and cozy, I most certainly did. We also ate Mongolian cuisine.

I'm ashamed to admit that the combination of chemo and my nerves left me with a short fuse that day. Kyle is always the only one around to bear the brunt of it. He is a pillar of strength, enduring the best and worst of me and all the changes that accompany both illness and medication.

I grew frustrated with the constraints of my body. It felt as if a thick fog settled over my memory. Suffering from insomnia, let me tell you getting one hour of sleep over a thirty three hour period will lead to occasional weeping for the healthiest person.

My annihilated immune system made me feel chilled me to the bone, always cold. Somehow, beneath all of this I knew there was strength within me.

Within just a few days, the second dose of chemo made me feel strong and rejuvenated. I weighed the most I have ever weighed in my life. For this I could only conclude this with a statement I've made and will continue to make, "You just can't win for losing."

I experienced new symptoms. Fear clutched me tightly while voicing them. I had a lingering fear that if I voiced what I was experiencing, others would confirm it and then it would become reality. Old habits die hard.

I was forced to look at how my life was impacting everyone around me. I had little control over the hurt they were feeling while watching me dwindle.

Kyle, my knight in shining armour was beside me day and night. Oddly enough, I still felt alone in my battle. I knew there were patients facing similar challenges, but nobody spoke of what the outcome would be. There was hardly any feedback about being terminal. Perhaps for them, voicing it would make it too realistic as well.

My hair began falling out near the end of October. Staring at a sink full of strands, I cried while drying my hair. Kyle wanted to shave my head, but I wanted to wait until it was coming out in clumps.

The doctors reviewed my progress since September, they were pleased. They set a date in early November to schedule preparations for the procedure.

Being so far from home, I looked forward to calls from friends and family. Absence really does make the heart grow fonder.

I found myself able to function at the most bizarre times, not the most logical. This, in a way, is the epitome of the very complex disease which is multiple sclerosis. Even in the late and terminal stages of my disease I was still surprised by some of the oddities from symptoms.

Also complex was the constant issues of trying to maintain our out of province coverage.

One day while having some issues putting on a shoe I gave up and began to cry.

Kyle lovingly reminded me, "You know, you can ask for help."

I was regaining balance and I was improving in other aspects of my abilities. I felt pride dressing independently in the morning.

I even walked a few steps on my own.

I was indebted to my body on my birthday. It was a good day, we got out of our room to get a coffee and tried a new lasagna that was being served at the coffee shop. We spent the evening watching baseball and I wouldn't have had it any other way.

I had to do another treatment before I could have my procedure. I was given injections to make my bone marrow rapidly produce more cells. I was informed this would be a painful process. This wasn't a lie.

On October 29 a beloved member of my family passed away. Of course I felt physical pain from my grief.

The next morning I saw doves outside my window. I called my mother and we shed a few tears about the sighting. The passing of my loved one encouraged strength and invoked motivation. I showered by myself within earshot of Kyle for the first time since August. Later on I climbed stairs, it was miraculous!

Financial issues weighed heavily on me and Kyle. Our funds were depleting and I felt like a burden. I scouted for donations from friends and family, hoping to relieve some of the strain from Kyle's bank account. I put my house and truck up for sale but nobody was interested. There were many people who said they would help, but it seemed they forgot as quickly as we hung up the phone.

The third step prayer from my program soothes a long day. It gives me great pleasure to share it with you.

The Third Step Prayer

"Life with Hope Higher Power,
I have tried to control the uncontrollable for far too long.
I acknowledge that my life is unmanageable.
I ask for your care and guidance.
Grant me honesty, courage, humility, and serenity,
to face that which keeps me from you and others
I give this life to you to do with as you will."

*NOVEMBER*

By November Kyle was not resting easily. We were both grateful to have 90% coverage for my medications. But with $7000 injections, the bill was still pricey.

The procedure was imminent. Even with his concerns, Kyle stood strong. Amazing, while dealing with his own inner turmoil, he still had the energy and patience to manage my upheavals.

The first ten days in November 2011 I made large accomplishments. I stepped over the edge of the tub without the use of my hands, and then I dressed myself. I walked daily, feeling stronger with each step. The more I accomplished on my own, the better my mood became. Ironically, Kyle and I were getting on each other's nerves.

November 3rd I had an appointment with Dr. Freedman for a final evaluation to qualify for the Hematopoietic Stem Cell Replacement (HSCT). That morning I was up before my alarm went off, anxious with anticipation. I could feel that my legs were quite shaky but I managed to get myself dressed and ready. There was so much on the line today, not so much with my [22]BMT team appointment, but with the MS evaluation. I was spooked. Kyle and I decided to have a coffee before my 8 o'clock appointment with the Hematology (BMT) team. I didn't walk at all prior to the test; I saved my energy for the MS

---

22    BMT: Bone Marrow Transplant

evaluation appointment. 7:45 am we headed across the street to the hospital to check in. I felt antsy and when we were the only ones left in the waiting area, I became nervous that they were leaving us out. My fingers were dancing a weird neurological twitch of repetition that I often do when feeling stressed. I rub my index finger nails on the pads of my thumbs and vice versa. It can become so tedious that I have cut myself before. Kyle took my hand, settling the activity. He made a wise crack of putting gloves on me again.

A nurse came and called us in.

She immediately began taking my specs, blood pressure, temperature, height and weight. When she was finished, she smiled and handed us both a piece of paper with my orders. The paper had information that told us where to be and when for the next 20 days starting on Remembrance Day. It was indeed a day to be remembered, no pun intended. Remembrance Day I would be admitted to the hospital where I would receive my first dose of Cyclophosphamide. They would keep me for 2 days to receive chemotherapy and fluids. The 2nd day they would teach Kyle and I how to self-administer the [23]Neupogen shots.

---

23    Neupogen is a man-made form of a protein that stimulates the growth of white blood cells in your body. White blood cells help your body fight against infection. Neupogen is used to treat neutropenia, a lack of certain white blood cells caused by cancer, bone marrow transplant, receiving chemotherapy, or by other conditions. Source: http://www.drugs.com/neupogen.html

I found this amusing because I didn't need any advice about how to give myself a needle. I have done it regularly for three years.

We were required to self-administer the shots in our room at the Rotel every morning.

Eight vials of blood were taken out of me and sent to infectious diseases. There it would be checked for every disease known to man.

After all this excitement we went back to our examination room to wait for [24]Dr. Bredeson. Dr. Bredeson is a brilliant doctor specializing in stem cell transplantation. He went over questions we had, including what Kyle should watch for when we returned to the Rotel. They discussed Kyle's anticipations for my recovery. Dr. Bredeson told Kyle that his expectations were too high. If Kyle lowered them, there was a better possibility he wouldn't be let down.

Afterwards, my pre-transplant advisor came back and handed us a book with 100 pages of information. There was so much information to read. Having all of this information at hand was wonderful. It was also a huge reality check of how BIG of a deal it was.

After receiving the book we headed upstairs for my MS evaluation, following was an appointment with Dr. Freedman.

The evaluation was the make or break of the transplant. There were many fearful days in my life, but this felt the scariest.

I walked with a walker, which by this point I had not done in a

---

24     Information Source: http://www.ohri.ca/profile/cbredeson

month. I had been using railings and pushing my wheelchair. I was nervous.

Marjorie pulled out a 4 wheeled walker. The one I was renting had 4 wheels as well, but it had automatic brakes that would make it stop if I leaned downward. The one Marjorie brought out was a normal walker, no special brakes, I was unsure of how I would fare. As it turned out, it wasn't as bad as I thought. My legs were a little wobbly to start off and I was glad they cooperated after a couple steps. I managed to walk 450 feet! The requirement was only 100. I did great! They even timed me for crap sakes!

They needed to see what my baseline was for the [25]EDSS scale, which is a method of measuring disability in multiple sclerosis. 1 was the best score you could have under the circumstances and 10 was death from MS. I was sitting at 8.5 when I arrived, now I was back to a 6. Thank the heavens!

It was also revealed after a full examination that my vision was back to 20/20. Dr. Freedman told me that the scarring on my left optic nerve is worse than my right; however, I do have it in both. I was already vaguely aware because I had lost my vision more in my left eye. I suffered many spells of double vision during my most recent relapse in Calgary.

---

25    The Kurtzke Expanded Disability Status Scale (EDSS) is a method of quantifying disability in multiple sclerosis. Source: http://en.wikipedia.org/wiki/Expanded_Disability_Status_Scale

They booked me in for an MRI of my brain and spine before cell producing started the following week. My left leg was still quite a bit weaker. Dr. Freedman had hoped that it would not be as 'hoppy' as it was but it wasn't so. It didn't matter now though, I had passed my evaluation and knew for sure that I would be receiving the procedure. All that was left was to exercise and keep practicing until my Neupogen infusions on November 11. I was booked for stem cell collection on November 22 and 23.

I found my nerves starting to calm the closer we got to getting everything underway. I was aware that there were major risks; the most severe being the loss of my life. I could hardly focus on anything else. As far as I was concerned my life was already over, and now I had to fight to save it. I was completely unaware of what the outcome would be, something inside me told me it was time to settle down and focus on the present. Stop worrying about the future.

As I improved my mobility, my inner organs began improving as well. They were beginning to function normally, all because I had some mobility. Poor Kyle was constantly soaking up my blood, shit and tears, literally.

I was plagued by muscle spasms. The pros of possibly getting well again were too good to let the cons of bothersome symptoms get the best of me.

MS is a tough opponent even at the best of times. One morning I awoke with a very painful MS hug. That same day, Kyle took me out in my wheelchair and placed me in front of a beautiful tree he found. He took a picture so we could remember, so I could remember the good from that day rather than the awful symptoms I had been suffering. This kind of thoughtfulness anyone would be lucky to encounter.

So much time spent away from loved ones caused me to reflect and reminisce. Through reminiscing there were fits of laughter and tears. Reflection left me grateful for having those memories, especially the good ones.

I was more aware of the kind and bad behaviours others displayed than ever before.

A friend of Kyles was raising money for us at work by passing a hat around collecting donations. By the time the hat reached him again, all the money put in had been stolen. I will never be able to fathom this kind of behaviour, from any person, for any reason.

The morning of November 10th was the worst day I experienced while in Ottawa. The Chemotherapy was starting to make me ill. I also had a messy accident in my bed that morning, one I had not experienced in a few months. My MS accidents had gotten better but this day it kept me on my toes. It was possible my MS was taking a stand, knowing its control over my life might soon cease.

I was building strength and practiced walking each day. Progressing so well, I didn't dare speak it out loud for fear I would jinx it.

I succeeded in walking 2000 feet. It was a great finale just before I started the most difficult part of my journey thus far. I never knew I had the capacity to be so excited and equally fearful at the same time.

In November, the 11th month, on the 11th day of 2011 at 11 am I was booked into the hospital for my stem cell collection regimen. They set up a bed for me in case I required a longer stay. Not long after arriving I was given an infusion of Cyclophosphamide. The following day they taught Kyle how to administer the infusions of Neupogen. On the third day I was given my first Neupogen injection and released to go home to the Rotel. I consoled myself through this by reminding myself that the procedure would be soon. Soon, I would be saved.

Kyle gave me the infusions for the next nine days. After those nine days, the following two days would consist of a two part stem cell extraction at the hospital.

Remarkably, with little rest I was still able to keep moving. I woke Kyle in early morning hours for showers after soaking diapers.

My strength was improving beyond my own comprehension. I loved it. If I didn't have to endure so many darn UTI's I would have been golden.

The bone pain was starting to present itself. The injections caused strange smells to emit from me. The smell was strong and acidic, similar to garlic.

One day I had an interaction from taking one of my many medications with my antibiotics. This resulted in more unnecessary suffering leaving me incredibly lethargic. It was awful but I learned a valuable lesson.

On November 22 I got up, showered, dressed and walked unassisted for 500 feet. During this milestone I battled a fever, because of my immune system issues I had to check my temperature four times a day thereafter.

After my walk it was time to start harvesting my blood for the stem cell extraction.

I was connected to an apheresis machine that ran my blood with a saline drip and an anticoagulant. The machine separated the cells within my blood. My right arm was hooked to the extraction machine while my left arm had a site for the re-entry of my blood and calcium. They kept me wrapped in warm blankets to prevent my blood from clotting.

The doctors were encouraging and the nurses were lighthearted, able to find ways to make jokes while assisting me using my bedpan. They were angels. If it weren't for their wonderful service my tale would be a lot bleaker.

After an entire day in bed and 24 litres of blood exchanged, I was tired but still able to get up and go for coffee with Kyle.

The entire process was repeated the next day. After my lips were tingling, my muscles vibrated and my fingertips went numb. I drank six glasses of milk because my calcium was depleted. On a good day, I won't drink a glass of milk by choice.

After a week of minimal movement I got up and walked 1000 feet behind my wheelchair. My muscles were tender from the calcium depletion. I felt lightheaded, dizzy and my hair follicles were throbbing in an agonising manner. Nobody told me that the process of losing your hair would be so painful. It was excruciating just to move my head in my sleep, brushing it was a nightmare.

On top of everything, Kyle's short term disability was refused. Kyle never held high regards for insurance companies. His told him that if he had stayed home he would have been covered for the time off work. They would allow him to distress over my absence alone at home. Since he came with me, the insurance company felt he was no longer distraught. We had to reapply and appeal for benefits before we used up all of his savings.

On the morning of November 25th I wept in the shower holding fistfuls of hair. In disbelief, I ran my fingers through my hair, pulling out more. I continued to do this hoping it would stop. Kyle collected me and settled me back into bed. When I regained my composure, the cutting and shaving began.

With a smooth head I noticed people's stares. It occurred to me that even while inside a hospital with a cancer ward, people still looked at you differently. Cancer patients came up to me and made nice remarks about my caps. I felt bad. I didn't understand their disease, I didn't have cancer. I had no way of voicing my feelings. The only thing I shared with these people was terminal suffering and hair loss. This also contributed to the loneliness I felt.

I missed my friends immensely, especially my female companions. Kyle, as incredible as he may be, was not so great or willing to sit and listen to me bitch and moan as my girlfriends would. Sometimes he gets tired of me and quite frankly, I do too.

Everyday seemed to be the same. We went for coffee and fruit runs, experienced good days and bad days, and practiced gaining strength.

My mother's MS was causing problems for her again and she was admitted into hospital for an infection. Being thousands of miles away, I felt helpless. It's ridiculous how MS can throw a wrench into lives over the simplest issues. I only have gratitude and admiration for my mother. It is because of my parents that I am so strong today.

I was confined to my room because I felt unwell but I was itching to be outside.

I found that shaving my head greatly diminished the pain felt in my follicles. The hardest part of losing my hair was when I was pulling out large clumps in the shower.

*DECEMBER*

The beginning of December, gifts were plentiful coming in through the mail. There were oodles of Christmas cards filled with cash. Teena sent me a Christmas care package consisting of a tiny tree with gifts. There were twelve gifts for the twelve days of Christmas, each one containing the items from the song. Sometimes there were challenging anagrams to keep me sharp, they were very special to my heart. It is one of the most thoughtful things anyone has done for me. It made the two weeks prior to Christmas bearable and brought much needed spirit to our Rotel room.

The 3$^{rd}$ of Dec was the first time I was able to step on an elevator in many years. My inability came from a resonating uneasiness with my lack of balance. Every time I got to the threshold of entering the elevator it felt like my brain would shut down. I wanted to step over the edge, but my body would freeze and not allow me to. It wasn't necessarily fear, as I said, it was more of an uneasiness that would translate into an irrational doubting of my own capabilities. Since that day I am no longer hindered by an elevator when the doors open.

Chemo caused extreme fatigue while my hair steadily fell out.

Kyle continued to shave the hair that hadn't fallen out yet. As he slid the razor across my scalp he noticed my hair coming out easily by the root.

I always looked forward to watching reruns of my favorite show, The Littlest Hobo.

I could walk unaided but getting out of bed was like towing a trailer without the truck.

On December 7$^{th}$ I received the transplant regimen, scheduled to take place on December 29, 2011. I would be admitted into hospital on December 19$^{th}$. Every day after until the 29$^{th}$ I would receive infusions of [26]Busulfan and more Cyclophosphamide, all in preparation for the transplant day. I would have a [27]PICC line placed in my arm the day I was admitted. Dr. Bredeson told Kyle and I that when I started on Busulfan we would know if Santa liked me or not. This drug is tremendously difficult on the system.

The hospital social worker gave Kyle paperwork for compassionate leave from work. The content was unnerving. There were questions asking, 'Is there a significant chance of death within the next twenty six weeks?' the reality was devastating.

Just after the first week in December we had a planning meeting which outlined the bone marrow transplant regimen. I was prescribed anti-seizure medications because I was having a three hour chemo infusion that had the potential to cause seizures.

After I received the chemo infusion and for the first time since arriving in Ottawa, I was able to cross the street that led from the hospital to the Rotel without fear.

December 10th I broke records with my recovery. I walked an astonishing 1.02 miles with my walker! My body filled with spasms, boy

---

26    Busulfan is used in combination with Cyclophosphamide as a conditioning agent prior to bone marrow transplantation, Busulfan can control tumor burden but cannot prevent transformation or correct cytogenic abnormalities. Source: http://en.wikipedia.org/wiki/Busulfan

27    A peripherally inserted central catheter (PICC) is a form of intravenous access that can be used for a prolonged period of time. Source: http://en.wikipedia.org/wiki/Peripherally_inserted_central_catheter

was I sore, but it was a result from progress. It is amazing how a poison like chemotherapy can produce such miraculous results.

My body was getting stronger and I could feel my MS fighting back. MS is a horrible disease to have, also horrid for those who have to support people bestowed with it.

I had continuous spasms and nerve sensations that felt like I was being stabbed by icepicks in my wrists. I could only endure the pain and pray that I would walk further each day. I fought my disease hard, surprised expressions on the nurses and doctor's faces from my progress only encouraged me. It gave me an invisible strength to push forward.

During all of this, Kyle and I were still mulling over paperwork, trying to get his compassionate leave from work sorted out. There was nothing compassionate about this aspect.

Speaking of compassion, December 17th is Kyle's birthday and I was feeling horrible this day. I couldn't even lift my legs on my own. I was fighting off infections and filled up to my nostrils with antibiotics. I completely forgot it was his birthday and slept the entire day away. He would drop subtle hints but it wasn't until I was lucid in the evening that it dawned on me. We ordered in and ate together while watching TV.

The following day I felt awful for sleeping through Kyle's day, we were lucky I was well enough to take an evening stroll.

I struggle with my memory often, when unable to remember a

game show brought me to tears, Kyle suggested that I exercise my brain. Practice mental activities to keep me sharp. I felt as sharp as a dull pencil. While playing these games we fought the entire horrible time. My mind was SO off that I would get unbelievably angry out of frustration.

When December 19, 2011 came around I had my PICC line surgically put into my right arm. It connected to the largest vein at the top of my heart. Having the surgery proved to be a difficult process for the surgeon and I. While he was inserting the line, my muscle kept going into spasms and kicking it out of place. I had to apply heat over the site four times a day to prevent blood clotting. The surgery was fatiguing, according to staff I was on enough meds I could have knocked out two horses, a small elephant and a midget for twelve hours. This was the exact description they used.

From the 20th to the 22nd I received doses of Busulfan over the course of three hours each time. I was scheduled to have four more two hour long infusions of chemo starting Christmas Eve.

Kyle decorated my room for Christmas, bringing in as much spirit as allowed. I was grateful to have any at all, Kyle alone would have sufficed.

On Christmas day I was unable to sleep due to the chemo induced menopause. I kept having horrible hot flashes. Gigantic, fluffy snowflakes fell outside my window, I was perfectly content. Kyle downloaded an angry bird's game for me and I was greatly entertained.

We knew now that Santa liked me. I survived the Busulfan treatment. My gratitude was overwhelming. In a couple of short days I would be undergoing a procedure that would possibly save my life.

I fell asleep with an excruciating MS hug only to awaken on December 26, 2011, Teena's birthday, barely able to breathe. I was greatly swollen from being filled with fluids and infusions.

On December 29th I had my procedure, the [28]hematopoietic stem cell transplantation (HSCT). The team showed up bright and early. I remember them rolling in silver canisters that sat in the middle of my room. The canisters hissed as each one was opened. The sound was liquid nitrogen being released and it was visible as it came out the top of the cans. I had two main lines connecting me to a large machine. I had one site in each arm; I was connected to five more lines when they connected me to the transplant machine. All these lines made showering challenging, more so for Kyle. Something I never believed possible was that laughing could be painful. It was excruciating and my Kyle has a wicked sense of humor. I wish I could say that the transplant by itself was more exciting. The preparations leading to the transplant held most of the anticipation. I lied there most of the

---

28    Hematopoietic stem cell transplantation (HSCT) is the transplantation of multipotent hematopoietic stem cells, usually derived from
bone marrow, peripheral blood, or umbilical cord blood. It may be
autologous (the patient's own stem cells are used) orallogeneic (the
stem cells come from a donor). Source: http://en.wikipedia.org/wiki/
Hematopoietic_stem_cell_transplantation

day waiting, and waiting for my life to be changed and in eight hours the transplant was complete.

When we were done, Linda Hamlin, the nurse who performed the transplant stood in doorway of my room. She stopped, turned, looked at me and said, "HAPPY BIRTHDAY FIONA!"

After they put in the final bag of cells, I was filled with Fentanyl and Dilaudid, two kinds of opioid medications. I wasn't fully conscious for a few days, and I thank the doctors for this because they know what they're doing. The pain would have been too much to bear. During these days I failed to blog and all my daily readers feared the worst.

Now all that was left to do was to wait and see if the procedure had worked in halting my disease from progressing any further. I am the 30th person to receive HSCT for multiple sclerosis, and the 4th person outside of the original study trial.

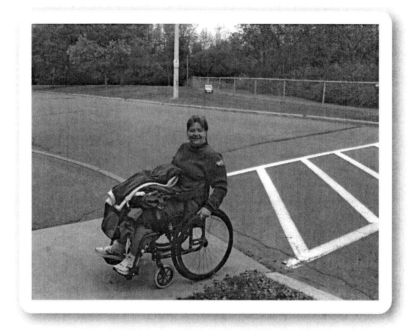

*Crossing the street to the Rotel*

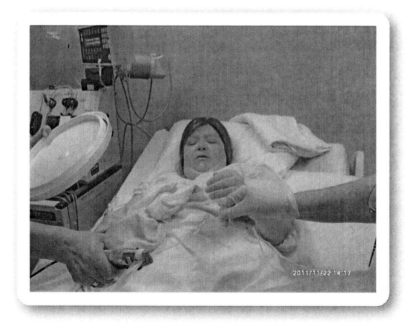

*Harvesting my cells*

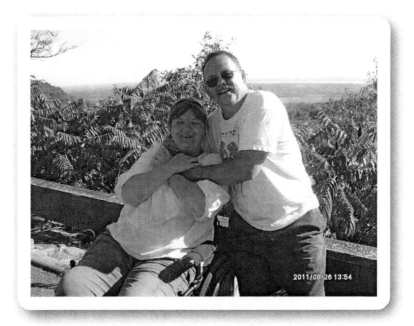

*Kyle and I overlooking the Ottawa Valley*

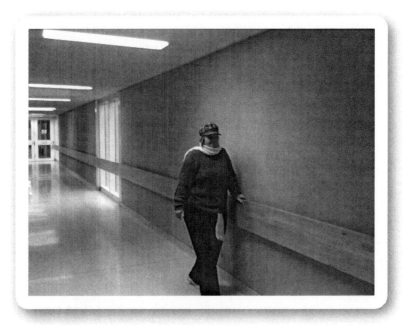

*Me practicing walking after Mitox in the hall*

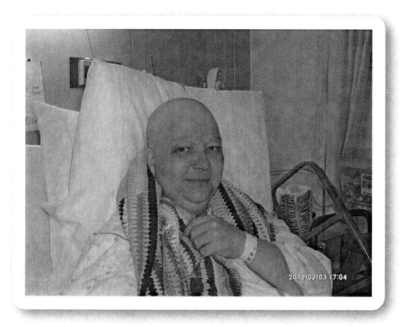

*Me without any hair, trying to keep warm*

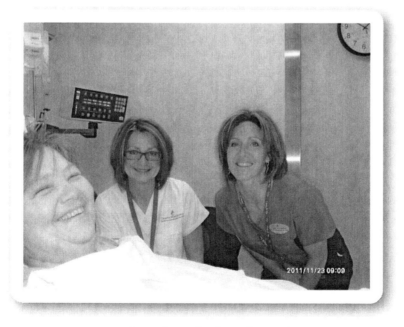

*My Canadian Blood Bank Angels*

Diagnosis: Multiple Sclerosis

PBSC Date: Nov. 22, 23, 2011          Harvest Date:
Cell Count: 3.96 x10^6 CD 34 enriched cells/kg    Cell Count:

## TRANSPLANT REGIMEN

*My transplant regime*

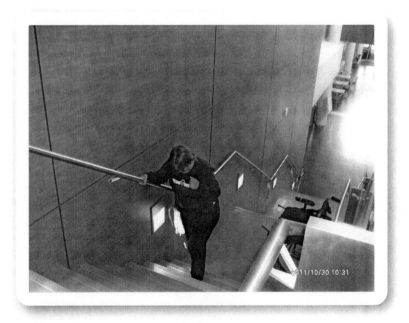

*Practicing walking up the stairs (2)*

198

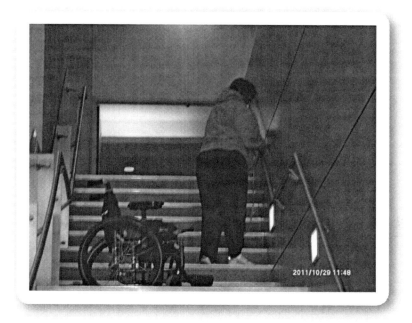

*Practicing walking up the stairs*

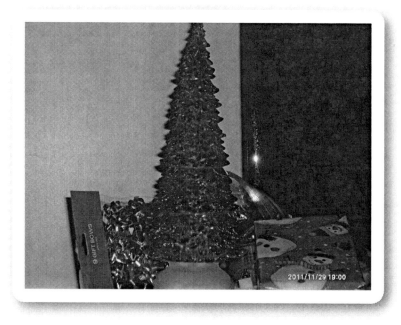

*The Christmas Tree and gifts Teena sent me*

# The First Year of Recovery

January 1, 2012 required a blood transfusion because my blood plate-lets were low.

Incredibly irritable and whiny, Kyle the saint, needed to take a breather from the frightfully snappy and whimpering Fiona. My pain stayed at intolerable levels forcing me to continue my heavy pain medications. Something I've never been enthusiastic about. My medications also caused me to have terrifying nightmares. My MS hugs were frequent. This made me reflect on the past and present, how I still channeled pain into anger, bestowing it on anyone around me. Poor Kyle was exhausted; the past five months were starting to weigh on him. I felt helpless and guilty.

On the bright side I reached another milestone, I could make it from the shower stall, to the toilet seat and then to bed. No trail of excrement and no diaper. If only my appetite flourished as my body seemingly was. With no desire to eat, I could hardly taste and this included my favorite foods. When I did manage to consume something, my digestion would produce spasms which would almost induce vomiting. As a result, I had a feeding tube placed into my nose, shoved down the back of my throat and into my stomach.

I loved the feeding tube. It made my life a little easier which made me feel pretty good. I was placed on a diet of ice chips for a few days; my stomach was quite torn up from the many treatments.

I developed large bruises in my armpits that reached to my inner upper arms. When platelets are low, blood is unable to clot and results in blood pooling beneath the skin. It looked worse than it was and it didn't bother me too much.

Looking around my room, seeing the equipment and personal items, I felt blessed. This was the room my life was saved in. There were no words for the gratitude I felt towards all of the angels who had entered and exited this room. Blessings were all around me, physically and spiritually, I could feel them all. An immense blessing is my family is a closer, stronger unit from coming together to help me endure the last five months.

Soon I started eating solid food again and continued my physio. Within a week my feeding tube was removed. My catheter was pulled out and I had to relearn how to urinate. This is quite the painstaking task for someone in my position. I had a commode beside my bed because the urgency of having to urinate, which now seemed foreign to me, was painful. It was difficult and heavy having to lift my swollen, fluid retaining legs out of bed. I can only ever take everything in stride, one day at a time, for whatever it may offer.

My truck and home that I had put up for sale were still not sold. Kyle put his own home for sale and it broke my heart that he was sacrificing more.

"A house is a house," he said when I expressed my feelings.

My health launched up and down like a yo-yo.

I battled low blood pressure, my low blood count made me feel faint often. I also had another bladder infection and endured excruciating headaches.

On the morning of January 18, 2012 after vomiting, I passed out while in the shower for 20 seconds. Thank God Kyle was assisting me at the time or I could have been seriously hurt. The very next day, while sitting in my commode after a day of physio, Kyle said I looked euphoric and was slow to respond. I lost consciousness for 15-20 seconds.

On January 21$^{st}$ I felt dizzy, fainting again in the shower. This time I lost consciousness for 15 seconds.

On the 23$^{rd}$ I lost consciousness in the shower yet again.

I fainted again the very next day during a rest period while attempting to do my sit and stand exercises. The same day, I used my commode only to feel that awful familiar dizzying feeling as I stood. I sat back down on the commode and fainted. I lost consciousness for 25 seconds while my eyes rolled in the back of my head. My fatigue was all encompassing; because I was fainting often I was not allowed to walk. I can't even begin to imagine how Kyle must have felt helplessly watching me in these episodes. I know how awful these experiences sound but my body was still adjusting to the procedure.

Almost a month post-transplant my taste buds were returning. The doctors were pleased with my progress. I was informed it would take months to rebuild my nervous system but it was something to look forward to.

*FEBRUARY 2012*

By the time February came along I could hardly believe so much time had passed. On February 2nd I was discharged from my unit to the rehabilitation unit. Kyle began spending his nights in the Rotel and this gave me separation anxiety.

I contemplated how life would be after arriving home. I had grown accustomed to being sick. The prospect of feeling and being healthy again made me feel exhilarated and terrified.

February 3rd was the first time I wore my clothes since Christmas Eve. My taste and sense of smell were taking longer than anticipated to return and emotionally, I was still very sensitive.

I was sick and tired of being sick and tired. That particular day was full of accidents and I was in dire need of a change of clothing. It was just a bad day and, after everything endured, these accidents made me want to quit. This made Kyle upset with me, he wanted me to stay strong and keep pushing. So I did.

Day later I could finally taste food again and it was delightful. I progressed in rehab and even my hair was showing signs of its itching return.

On Valentine's Day I was flat broke, unable to afford a gift for Kyle.

After weeping this woe to a nurse she very stealthily snuck in some chocolates and a book wrapped in towel. She knew how important it was for me that Kyle have a nice Valentine's Day too. Small acts of kindness like this stand out to me more than anything. It reminds me of how beautiful the world can truly be. On top of a wonderful Valentines, Kyle and I had the pleasure of meeting a Border collie named Liam, visiting patients in the hospital. I love animals more than people so this was a nice treat.

Having good days meant bad ones were due. They came while my emotions were erratic, leading me to cry over menial things. Still battling a damned infection, the unknown bug extended my stay another two weeks.

Kyle always sees the bright side. I'm forever indebted that he does during our trying periods. He reassured me we were better safe than sorry.

I took oral antibiotics, then intravenous antibiotics and then I received three bottles of [29]IVIG which is intravenous immunoglobulin. A blood product administered intravenously. It contains the pooled, polyvalent, IgG antibodies extracted from the plasma of over one thousand blood donors. It is a very pricey treatment.

After more brain scans, I was transferred to a medical daycare unit.

There, Kyle was taught how to administer intravenous antibiotics for me.

I suffered severe bowel issues and the hospital tested to make sure I didn't contract a nasty bug called C. Difficile. Thankfully, I didn't.

I had 21 prescriptions and even after 90% drug coverage the bill was still over $300. This is a lot to pay when you're being broke. We managed with help from friends and family, and Kyle was an excellent nurse.

On February 24th I was released from the hospital back to our Rotel room. I was supposed to be discharged a day prior but I developed a – yes you guessed it – a UTI!

I was held for another 24 hours because of the fever that surfaced. I had mixed emotions about returning to the Rotel. I knew Kyle was an excellent caregiver but I had reservations about my progress, after all, it had a habit of being short lived.

---

29     Source: http://en.wikipedia.org/wiki/Intravenous_immunoglobulin

*MARCH 2012*

Coming into March Kyle and I were having issues with our insurance. It is incredibly difficult to maintain insurance from another province. We were denied extra funding from a 'Little Angels' program that had assisted us with our living expenses. It felt like we had finally exhausted our resources, from all of our begging and borrowing.

Money problems lead to conflict in the healthiest relationships and Kyle and I were starting to bicker.

I think we were at each other's throats because we were stuck as the only company for one another too long. It was starting to lose its appeal. This with financial strains was a recipe for conflict.

Anger proved to be a reliable motivator. My anger fuelled me to walk well and gain extra distance. Even while pissing me off, he still encouraged me to progress.

My hair began growing again and I liked running my hands across the stubble. My new nails were growing under my old ones as well. It looked neat and there was no pain involved. What was important was keeping the old nails from hooking on anything and tearing off. I had been following a ladies blog in the UK who ended up losing most of her fingers due to infection from her nails ripping off too soon. By the time they were nearing half grown in Kyle figured out that crazy glue was the answer. He crazy glued my old nail to my new nail every day or every second day until they were close enough for me to clip them. My old nails had been weak and chipped easily. Remarkably, the new nails that I have now are hard and healthy.

I was experiencing symptoms and it was hard to decipher whether they were from my MS or from the chemo. Only time would tell.

My memory is no good when recalling difficult times. I think as a defense mechanism, to an extent, I willfully forget everything bad that happens to me. It is hard for me to remember a really bad day. I can only accurately relay my story to you through reading my daily blogs and hospital records.

I made some very productive realizations during this time. One of them was that, 'my body will always be the boss; I just need to pay attention.' This was easier to say than acknowledge – but awareness helps.

I was plagued by infection after infection, luckily this is not new territory, and I'm persistent. I continued to progress through the ailments with physio and IVIG infusions.

For the first time in a few years I weighed less than 200 pounds, it was elating. In the past, every time I became strong enough to battle my weight I would end up disabled, or on steroids or chemo.

The tension between Kyle and I was thickening. My antibiotics were not working. Tests showed I was fighting three different bugs and now, blood clots. Kyle started administering IV antibiotics every four hours for me. Kyle gets annoyed when I am lethargic. His intentions are only good when he wants me to get up and stay motivated.

But I just have bad days, sometimes more often than not. Sometimes I need to dwell before I can climb out of it.

I am grateful I have people who can relate to me, even if it is because they suffer from the same disease. It's important to have someone who can empathize and relate to you on a personal level. Kyle knows me well but because he doesn't have MS, he will never truly know. We MS patients have an unspoken bond which ties our suffering together.

I was doing exponentially well in comparison to before the transplant. I still suffered dizzying episodes and fatigue, but everything seemed to be improving. My progress was at a severely glacial pace, but I could feel it. The doctors felt it was a quicker pace than expected, so I had to be grateful for this. You won't be surprised to know that I was battling that blasted UTI the entire month too, periodically suffering from a fever and aches here and there. Even still to this day, it's been the only thing consistent with my health.

*APRIL 2012*

By April I felt much better. I couldn't wait to go home. I was so done with the hospital, miraculous as they had been; I missed my friends and family. We booked our flight home for April 17, 2012. Excitedly, I overstepped my place to book our flight home. My hematology team booked to see an infectious disease specialist before we would be allowed to leave. I decided to push my luck one more time. If he did say I wasn't well enough to go home, flights be damned I'd have been staying. Luck was on my side this time, my appointment was at 9 and our flight was at 2. This couldn't have been a better motivator for me to get my poop in a group.

I felt full of life and I was thriving. I began shipping my belongings back home. I had accumulated quite a bit over the last 8 months.

I was beyond thankful to be alive when just a year prior the outlook was not so good. Just a year prior my family and I were making arrangements for my death.

Ready to make leaps and bounds, Kyle kept me on a cautious leash. He knew me well enough to know I could ruin everything by overdoing it. His first priority is and will always be to keep me healthy.

I was diagnosed with 'Pseudomonas aeruginosa cystitis', which is basically a difficult way of saying, "recurring urinary tract infections". I'm sure this meant more work for Dr. Baverstock, my urologist back home.

The evening before we flew home, we shared a home cooked dinner with Joan and Neil. As I sat at the dinner table, my friends conversing joyously around me, I had to take a moment. I reflected on the struggles and miracles of my time spent in Ottawa. I looked at all the work I had put in during my stay and thought of all the work that still awaited me. A future I could look forward to.

## HOME AT LAST

We flew into Calgary and spent the night at a hotel before commuting home. Ralph picked Kyle and I up from our hotel in the morning and took us for breakfast where my friend Trysh joined us. They were both very excited to have me home. It was a blessing to be reunited with my dearest friends after so much time had passed.

It wasn't long before the MS clinic was calling me to come in. After returning home I had two doctors' appointments the following day and two more in that same week.

I also had a new doctor, one who had studied my families MS gene pool.

Although happy to be home, the loss of my independence weighed heavily on me. It was easy to be positive because I was alive, but it dampened my mood knowing that I still had relied on others. It would be a 6-12 month wait just to get my license back.

I used my walker everywhere I went and it seemed promising I could retire my wheelchair. My legs were shaky and my feet were sore and swollen. These were repercussions after a productive day.

It occurred to me that I was delusional about my recovery. I believed once I was home all would be well and restored. Nothing in my life has ever been that easy.

When I did try to relax I felt the pressures of everything that needed to be done. I had an overwhelming amount of paperwork that needed my attention.

On April 21, 2012 I showered and dressed myself. I went outside and stood on my deck, eagerly awaiting my friend to pick me up to take me to a meeting.

Having the ability to do this, shower, dress myself and stand outside, was a Godsend. After arriving home from the meeting I sat down and began to sort through the paperwork – this lead to a mini meltdown. Hadn't I done enough already? I could hardly fathom how I had so much more to do. It was never-ending.

There were more meltdowns to follow too.

One morning my aunt called. You would have thought the house was burning down from the way I was wailing over not being able to find a pair of pants.

I pondered aloud, questioning when my sanity would return, Kyle predicted it would be a few months – I believed it was a good possibility it might have never been there to begin with.

My mind was still foggy, one morning I rattled off about an aloe vera plant that had been cut. I thought it was dying. I had completely forgotten that the plant was used for an array of healing purposes. When I remembered I felt like an idiot. I was aware that the procedure had some cognitive side effects and it wasn't overly upsetting, it was just something else I would have to get used to. Along with all of the other minor and severe symptoms I was experiencing.

On one of our trips into the city for appointments I made plans to meet with my grandparents. The plans fell through because Kyle and I didn't have enough time to squeeze them into our schedule. When this happened I had the very content understanding that this was okay. Neither my grandparents, nor I would be going anywhere anytime soon. A statement I couldn't make a year ago!

When I saw my mother for the first time since before I left for Ottawa, we shared a moment. We shed a few tears at the sight of each other.

With a loving embrace, instead of saying, "welcome home" or, "I love you!" She simply looked me over and said, "Wow! You have hair!"

I spent an entire day with my parents. My mother helped me sort my tax papers and then we played floor curling. I walked unaided while playing the game. While at the 50+ Curling Club, I got the opportunity to thank all of the people who had generously donated funds to Kyle and I while we were in Ottawa.

April 25th I was at a local A&W chain restaurant, they were having a penny drive to fundraise for MS. It was quite an event. There were radio announcements, the ladies from the MS society were present to show their support and reporters were on the scene.

Later that day, I had a neuro exam. Dr. Pearson was on vacation so I met with her covering neurologist, Dr. Jarvis. I walked into my appointment using Kyles arm to balance. He watched me walk 25 ft. unaided, then back and forth again. Dr. Jarvis took a video with his phone of my miraculous recovery.

On April 27$^{th}$ Kyle went to see his doctor to check up on his own health for the first time in a year.

I was delighted and overwhelmed by all the visits from friends and family.

One day while visiting with my mother's friend, she paid me the best compliment I have ever received, "you are your mothers' daughter" she said.

I have boundless love, respect and admiration for my mother, the compliment brought tears to my eyes.

I found myself reminiscing often of what the year prior consisted of. I was in awe with the milestones I had crossed. I could see the astonishment of being alive reflected within the eyes of my friends and families.

Slowly regaining energy, I shocked myself daily with my productivity.

In May I walked all throughout Costco, something I never dreamed I would be able to do again. That same day was the first time since before the procedure I got to see Teena and Ann. Tears were rolling upon seeing Ann. We had a nice catch up and I couldn't find words to express the immeasurable gratitude I felt just for knowing her.

Kyle and I began looking at houses, I couldn't shake the crappy feeling that came with our lives resuming to a level of normalcy. It was similar to Ottawa in the manner that we had created another schedule. I craved more excitement than the mundane day to day routine offered. Really looking at it, the day to day was still incredible, I was doing laundry, showering independently, sweeping, mopping, dusting and loading the dishwasher all while performing daily exercises. Leave it to me to be unsatisfied.

I began experiencing some issues with sleeping; I wasn't sure whether it was due to the nightmares or the bowel or bladder issues. Not long after I also noticed my vision faltering a bit. This required a visit with my Neuro-Ophthalmologist Dr. Costello. She worked with my entire medical team when she worked in Ottawa. It brought me great pleasure to chat about everyone when I saw her.

On May 7th Kyle had his first day back at work and I was comfortable being home alone again. I was reaching milestones daily. One milestone, I walked with a laundry basket in both hands, menial to many, substantial for me. Steadily progressing, after tiring and eventful days I still walked with the assistance of my cane or walker. I was learning my body's limits, taking it easy when necessary to avoid getting worn out. Now that time was back on my side I had the patience to do so.

Mother's day was another day to be grateful for. I spent the day with my parents, Teena, my nephew Michael and Kyle. My mother innocently inquired as to what we were all doing on this day a year prior.

My response was, "hospital mom."

On this day a year ago, my family was drawing up funeral plans for me along with a DNR (do not resuscitate) form. It was still a raw subject that left an air of uneasiness we all felt, but still, I think it made us all the more grateful.

Kyle and I searched properties and mid-May we found a beautiful home outside of Trochu, AB. It sat on 10 rolling acres of prairie land with decks facing east and west. It would be perfect for watching the sunrise in the morning and the sunset in the evening. Just a couple days after putting in an offer, it was accepted on the condition that one of our houses sold quickly. This deal fell through, neither house sold.

The month of May will always be a difficult month for me since my accident. The most horrendous things that have happened to me in my life happened in May. Whenever May 21st rolls around I am reminded of that fateful day. Hit by the blasted drunk driver which triggered my malignant disease to surface. Kyle was well aware of the emotional rollercoaster I would be on when I got home. I still had some resonating denial about my recovery, sometime bad days felt like relapses. To top everything off I was having some GI (gastrointestinal) issues again. No matter how many times I defecate myself, it never gets easier and always leaves me in tears.

One afternoon I decided to take a walk by myself. It didn't take long for Kyle to pull up with the truck and see if I required a ride yet. I walked as far as my legs allowed me, almost a full kilometre. It sucked out every ounce of energy I had and Kyle had to lift my legs into the truck. By the time we were home I was able to walk up the ramp and into our house.

May 21$^{st}$ Kyle and I took a drive to see a property we really liked.

On our way back home we headed southbound on the highway when Kyle and I saw what was about to happen. He was reacting as I was yelling "Kyle!"

A young woman in a little red car was pulling out from a stop sign onto the highway. Kyle slammed on the brakes and swerved left. I watched in shock and I knew there was no stopping what was about to happen. Kyle swerved so we didn't T-bone the woman completely but we made contact. We slammed into the front quarter panel of her car. We hit so hard that my side of the truck smashed sideways with her driver's side before we both went flying to either side of the road. We stopped in the east ditch and she landed in the west ditch. The airbags blew on initial impact; this terrified me because I've never been in an accident with airbags. The sound is explosive. I touched the dashboard airbag, desperately trying to figure out what was happening.

I was yelling at Kyle, "the truck is on fire, omg the truck is on fire."

Kyle, calm as ever said, "It's okay, it's just the airbags. They're hot from the chemical compounds."

Still panicked, I began to settle myself. Doors were opening and there were people everywhere. I got out and once I was on the ground my body went to hell. Kyle ran over to check the girl we hit, she had glass in her head from the shattered windows, but she was okay. Kyle checked me over and two off duty nurses approached us. They had watched the entire accident.

The girl we hit was quite young, only 19 or 20. I felt bad for her, having such a bad accident so early in life. She was hurt worse than Kyle or I. If Kyle hadn't swerved she would definitely have died.

Both of our vehicles were written off.

The seatbelts left quite a few bruises but our injuries were minor. We were all transported to the hospital by ambulance where we were assessed in trauma and shipped to the emergency room. After we were given the go-ahead to leave, the parents of the young woman who collided with us gave us a ride to a hotel.

I was beside myself, incredulously seven years to the day I was in another car accident. The following day we obtained a rental car, drove to my totalled car and cleared out all our belongings. I didn't have extra medication with me and, because of this, now I always carry an extra day's meds with me. We filled out all the necessary paperwork and went home. We made it safe and sound, in reasonably good health and quite exhausted. The next day I glanced at a photo we had taken of the wreck. I couldn't help but feel convinced that God really did intend for me to be here.

With the accident and preparations to sell the house, there was no shortage of priorities.

Training for the upcoming MS walk I managed to walk a full mile and climb a very tall set of stairs. Kyle's brother was getting married and his wedding was on the horizon. We went to the mall to find formal attire and I squeezed into a size twelve. I almost fell over, literally and figuratively. It was nice to see the weight was starting to come off.

I missed Teena's graduation for her Bachelor of Arts degree, this disappointed me greatly. After her graduation, my parents came to our house to pick up a wheelchair they had lent me before the procedure. It was a lengthy drive home so they spent the night. When my mother went to the spare bedroom she was delighted she could get into the bed effortlessly. I was witnessing my mother's milestones too. Five years ago the beds height had been too tall for her to climb into.

For the first time in 8 months I slept for 11 hours straight in the first week of June. I was also walking completely unaided. I shaved my legs for the first time in a lengthy stretch of time. Previously, I wasn't allowed to shave because if I cut myself, the risk of infection was far too risky for my crap immune system I met someone who had also applied for the transplant but was denied because they were not 'sick enough'. Just another reminder of how very grateful I am to be alive today.

Things were beginning to resume to a blissful state of normalcy. Kyle was busy working on the house and working at his job. I was busy progressing, happy when he had the time to participate in a walk with me.

One day while Kyle and I were walking we ran into one of my first physio therapists, Evelyn. She helped me learn to walk after my first paralysis in the fall of 2009. She and Calvin worked with me for six months. She was personal trainer I hired after my first paralysis. If it weren't for Evelynn, I would never have been able to go back to work. Funny thing is, when she approached us I did not recognize her until she hugged me and said who she was. It all came rushing back. She had moved away and it was pure coincidence we ran into her. She was only in town so her little one could visit with grandma. This is a prime example of how God puts people in my path at the right time. My life is like a jigsaw puzzle, piece by piece, it eventually all fits into place.

Kyle and I continued attending meetings together. I am thankful for the program, grateful it inspired spirituality. As well as the realization that I was not giving myself enough credit for coping with the past two years of my life.

In the following days I was scheduled to have an MRI of my brain and spine. The doctors wanted to see if the BMT had any definitive results. I also found that my IVIG treatments were having some adverse side effects. I felt dizzy, sometimes while moving my head it felt as if it would blow right off – this was coupled with an aberrant inability to stay awake, feeling incredibly lethargic.

My poor mother got wound up whenever I blogged about my 'off' days. I call her every day to reassure her, also so we can share our downfalls and accomplishments. There are many days she does amazing. One day she was all giddy because she and dad had made cookies for the first time in twenty five years. Their strength and ability sometimes shames me into doing more. I love them both so much for how well Teena and I have turned out. When I get overwhelmed my family is a reminder that I am not alone. As unfortunate as having this disease is, I am very fortunate that my family understands my battle and can empathize with my trials.

Before the procedure I fought change hard. I'd always be devastated when things didn't go as planned. My second chance at life has made it easier for me to accept things as they are.

On June 15th my dearest Ralph was reported missing. I was saddened he was absent for my small milestones. Like sitting on a yoga ball, or being able to chew gum for the first time in months. I wanted to call him and tell him all I was accomplishing. I think the need to call him was stronger because I knew he would not answer the phone. The stress of his disappearance weighed heavily on my body. When his daughter, Angie's birthday rolled around one week later I could hardly stand to think of the pain she was feeling. Kyle kept me moving along but I had a hard time sleeping. I would wake up talking to Ralph.

On June 26th I received my seven yearlong settlement cheque for my accident. It was from the initial crash that made my body spiral downhill into an MS nightmare. The man who had hit me that night had passed away so the Saskatchewan government would be suing the vehicles owner; he was liable to return their money.

Kyle and I drove to my lawyer's office in the city to pick up the cheque. While driving home we passed by the accident location in the industrial part of the city. Ironically, just meters away from where I was hit there was a road blockage because of another accident that had taken place. I hoped they fared better than I.

Things were looking up, after a bathroom break in Coleman I came out to find Kyle standing in front of a bulletin board. He was staring at a posting for puppies and it only took a moment before we were calling the number. Within a couple hours we were bringing home 6 week old Itchy. Itchy proved to be inspiring and kept me company on my morning walks. The first walk I took her out on I was able to walk completely unaided, with no walker or cane. Itchy became an admired companion in our daily lives. Itchy truly helped me through the dark days. She needed to be let out, trained and cared for. This motivated me on days I didn't want to get out of bed or off the couch. In many ways I wouldn't have come as far as quickly as I did without her.

Even with the settlement cheque and new puppy, Ralph was still in the back of my mind.

Kyle and I walked into a store that Ralph and I had frequented together. As we were concluding our shopping I said, "Are you ready Ralph?"

It was a disappointment I feared that I would have to get used to.

During moments like these the loss of Ralph becomes painfully clear. I remember the last time I saw Ralph, the last moment we shared.

Two weeks before I got the call saying he had been reported missing was the last time I saw him. I have another friend who resides close by Ralph's place and this is where Ralph and I often met up. Ralph lived on the third floor on an apartment and he was concerned I would get hurt venturing up the stairs.

I would insist I could handle the climb and he would say, "Fiona I am too frail. If something happened to either one of us then what?" He was right, always the wisest of the pair.

After meeting, we drove and parked at Edworthy Park down along Memorial Drive in Calgary. The Bow River runs along the park and there is a little restaurant that serves burgers and such. Ralph and I grabbed ice cream and chatted as we walked along the river. It was the first time since being home that I got to spend some quality alone time with him. We exchanged stories about what we'd been up to while I was away. We caught up and enjoyed the rest of the afternoon together. I often wonder now if he knew this would be our last encounter.

On June 29th I paid my parents back the $18,000 I owed them. Paying them back felt like one very large breath of fresh air. Owing them money and having that amount accumulate over the years made me feel I was choking on the debt. It made me sick to my stomach to know that I owed them that much money when they had their own financial struggles. After I paid the government the $23,000 I owed and my lawyer took his cut, I had a whopping $1000 leftover for myself.

On Canada Day I ended up in the emergency room with excruciating pain in my kidneys, which was followed by a trip to the pharmacy for antibiotics for a bladder infection. It didn't take long for me to bounce back again though, just a few days later I was practicing not wearing diapers in the evening. I am pleased to say I had some success!

Cooking one evening, I phoned my mother because it had been a long time since I had cooked a stew. I needed her assistance so I didn't screw it up. I'd been on the outside of living my life for so long that the things I loved to do seemed no longer in my reach.

Days passed and I started feeling weak again. I knew the culprit would be a UTI. I've stated how much I despise taking pain medication. The pain I was experiencing made me give in and take a Dilaudid.

My vision acted up too and I recalled a warning from the doctors. They said the first year and a half after my transplant things could happen with little to no explanation at all. These unexplainable incidents happened more than I could have anticipated. The right side of my body would act up feeling very tight resulting in me not being able to put much weight on it. There was a day I felt so nauseous and faint I called Kyle home from work for the first time. The doctors could find nothing wrong, no explanation. These are the times I needed to let go and let God.

On the topic of no explanation, our sweet little angel Itchy appeared to have a disagreeable attitude within her we weren't aware of. The first time I left her alone she completely destroyed our house. She defecated everywhere and even managed to pull down the blinds. She quite literally busted everything she could get her cute little muzzle on.

By mid-July it had already been a year and a half since I sat in the driver's seat of a vehicle. I could hardly stand it. I longed for the freedom to get up and go anywhere and do anything by myself. Healthy people often take this for granted. I reminded myself to be grateful for the simple things, like being able to roll over or get out of bed, feed myself and move all my extremities. While sifting through my paperwork I came across a small stack of invoices from hospitals in the US. I couldn't believe I worked while being so ill.

I was given more tests to see if information was being relayed to my brain properly. I also had my vision tested. All of these tests were imperative for me to get my license back.

The antibiotics for my UTI were not working. The tension of not feeling well again caused Kyle and me to bicker over theories why my body was uncooperative. The doctors tried a new antibiotic hoping it would relieve my symptoms. I experienced difficulties with swallowing. Everything I ate had to be choked down with a glass of water. I experienced lapses in my short-term memory, bouts of forgetfulness and minor confusion to follow. The doctors confirmed that these symptoms were from the transplant. On the upside, I did receive a call from Marjorie letting me know that the test results from my MRI revealed no new lesions. The news helped me with some of my fears of hopelessness that my health might be failing again.

It made me contemplate the actual severity of my disease and how ignorant I had been to it. I hadn't gone into remission once since being diagnosed in 2005. Any progress made was medically induced. My health would fail as soon as the medications were finished, if they had any affect at all. The most amazing revelation of the last two years was that I stayed alive long enough to have my transplant, halting my disease from progressing further.

On July 29th Kyle and I drove to Moosejaw, SK to attend his brother's wedding. This was the first time I met all of Kyle's family. He had disappeared from their lives, other than phone calls after we got together. It was another moment of intense gratitude, to be able to partake in such a joyous occasion. The event certainly took the attention away from me.

Only days later, my UTI returned a third time. I had just completed a third round of antibiotics. I noticed the symptoms were not as severe as before the transplant, before they always resulted in a hospitalization.

August 10, 2012 was my 21st sobriety birthday. It is an important date for me because without my sobriety I surely would not have made it tell my story today.

My sister sent me a card that read:

*"This is not 20 and 21, but much more accurate is Twenty- WON!! Last year the doctors did not think you would see one more, but they do not know you!"*

She could not have said it any better; she has such a wonderful way with words. I LOVE YOU Teena.

It was a terrific sobriety celebration with friends, laughter, love and cake. The greatest part of this night was catching meteors shooting across the sky with Kyle. Kyle and I finally got to have the very first date he had planned for us, a night of star gazing.

Still rather worn down by the end of the day, Kyle had me lie down for a rest in the afternoon to prepare for the long night ahead. He packed up lawn chairs, blankets and coffee, all this for comfort while we sat perched up on the side of a mountain well above the town of Sparwood, BC. He had his binoculars and telescope at hand so we could check out what lay beyond the stars. He's very technical while I'm merely a simpleton. Even though I knew it was a meteor shower, I watched innocently and wished on all those shooting stars. Astronomy enthralls Kyle. He becomes animated, with a childlike innocence when he talks about the sky. I learn so much from his enthusiasm. In moments like this we completely merge together as one.

A few days later I had a dental appointment and this made me excited. Because of the risk of infection I had been restricted from seeing a dentist by my BMT team. I required more antibiotics to have this appointment, and would for the rest of my life. But I was allowed to go and all the merrier for it. I had Vicki pick me up to bring me to my appointment and she brought her children, Natalie and Nathaniel with her. I was told when leaving Ottawa that it would be at least a year before I would be able to be in contact with children. My immune system was going strong so I wasn't overly concerned. It's not like they could give me a UTI, which is the only infection I have real issues with. I was happy to watch the children play with Itchy.

A couple days later I vacuumed my home for the first time in 5 years. This was an amazing feat for me while cleaning my house. Of course the next day my body was shouting that I had overworked myself. I rested the entire following day, wondering what else I might be able to accomplish.

Around this time I was asked to speak on a panel with other's that had the stem cell treatment for a webcasting radio station for MS. There was a difference between them and I though. They had what's called a Non-Myleo Blood Stem Cell Treatment without chemotherapy, whereas mine was a Hematopoietic Stem Cell Replacement. I was informed I should always call mine a procedure, not a treatment, treatments are repeated processes. I was greatly honoured by this and it wasn't long before Kyle and I were asked to do an interview.

Not much time passed when I acquired a severe bladder infection that caused excruciating discomfort and unbearable joint pain. Having a particularly bad attitude this day, I was angry with myself for having the transplant. This pain was seemingly worse than anything I had endured before. I tried to convince myself that I would already be out of my misery if I had not gone to Ottawa. This is kind of thought process is unproductive and borderline insane but they are legitimate feelings when enduring too much for too long. I had a better attitude after talking with my doctor and Kyle. Attending a meeting helped immensely too.

There was a lot to be joyous for. I attended my parent's 49th wedding anniversary, a well-deserved event. Kyle and I attended his company's gold golfing tournament and I won $50 for the longest female drive on the 7th hole. Golfing was a great challenge and I didn't fall once. It's quite impressive really. I accomplished all of this while battling a UTI.

In tune with my newfound abilities I booked a driver's test for the beginning of October in Lethbridge with Drive Able. The test would consist of both physical and cognitive analysis to determine whether I was fit to have my license back.

Unfortunately the day I booked my test also happened to land on the last day of my four month stretch of antibiotics. I grew frightfully nervous that my body would fail me as it often did when medications were finished. My subconscious anxieties were apparent in my dreams. I had nightmares I was sick all over again. Nursing staff were rolling my body in bed to prevent bed sores and I was fully paralyzed. I woke up terrified and it took hours to return to sleep. While I laid awake waiting for sleep to return, thoughts of Ralph would surface making it more difficult.

Kyle traded his manual truck in for an automatic one so I would have a vehicle to drive in the future. With the new truck he drove me out to a back logging road where there was no traffic. I had an examination for a driver's test in a couple weeks so we were testing my driving skills. I needed to see if my nerves were settled enough to drive. I did amazing. I had no doubts I would receive my licence back. If I was lucky enough, maybe even my class one. I was betting that everything would fall back into place and I was consumed with joy.

By the end of September I finished most of my Christmas shopping. I could hardly contain my excitement that this year I would be able to wrap gifts while listening to carols. I actually took a picture of the first present I wrapped and decorated, I was so proud. It would also be the first year in two years I could afford gifts. Before, I was so broke I had to use the food bank just to feed myself.

Around this time I started going to a class at the gym organized by Alberta Health Care for people with advanced illness. Here I met three beautiful souls also plagued by MS. It turns out one of the members knew of me before I had even met her. She read my blog and had been praying for me for months. We measured our accomplishments together. Mine would have blown my doctors out of the water. I was jogging with my walker, not even tripping over my own feet. I successfully jumped which is something I hadn't done in many years.

The real estate market in Coleman was slow. If you can believe it, Kyle and I's houses were not selling. It wasn't until the beginning of October, one day before my driver's test that we were preparing for our first viewing in two months. Even if it turned out to be a waste of time, I was too excited about my driver's test.

I am pleased to tell you I passed my test with flying colors. The instructor even stated, "When you get stronger, call my office and I will hire you as an instructor."

My license was reinstated and you can imagine my shock when the clerk at the registry asked me if I wanted my Class 1 back. You bet your ass I did. Also remarkable, I didn't need to have another driver's medical for 5 years. Since being diagnosed I've had to do the testing annually.

For the first time in years I was able to go out to our truck, hop in it and drive myself to town to attend a meeting. I got in, cranked up the music and sang all the way uptown and back! I cannot explain this joy. I had not been on my own in a very, very long time.

I can recall an afternoon, only days after my newfound freedom. I sat outside, feeling the warmth of the sun shining on my face. I was completely content. The sun would disappear behind a cloud and the temperature would drop. When I think of putting such a simple thing into perspective, it amazes me how sometimes my life and mood can do the same thing. This metaphor made it easier for me to make it through the next day because, no matter what, the sun will always shine, through stormy clouds and after dark nights, it will always return.

On October 14th I felt 'off', it was the first time I had to sit while showering in a couple of weeks. Kyle and I went to the hospital and when I checked in I saw my doctor through the window in the emergency room.

He took one look at me and said, "What are you doing here?"

I just gave him a look and I knew he could read my mind. I gave a urine sample for the umpteenth time and when they dipped the test strip, shock! Shock! It was infected!

They sent it away to be cultured. They sent me home exhausted with another week's worth of antibiotics. I was in disbelief how this infection could continue to attack me, wearing my body down a little more every time. It rouses underlying fears that one day I won't be healthy enough to combat one pesky infection. I wasn't going to let this hold me back though, not when I was regaining my independence.

One morning I drove Kyle to work then headed into town for a physiotherapy appointment at 11. After my appointment I had lunch with some of my girlfriends. This day felt like a normal day, like who I used to be before my disease took the reins. It was truly blissful to be out by myself, doing everything on my own, on my own schedule.

Soon after, unexplainable symptoms crept up again and it felt like Charlie horses multiplied by ten. It was a gnawing pain in my calf muscle and in the thin muscle that runs down the side of my shin to my ankle bone. I paid close attention to every step I took that day, for fear they would start spazzing and I would end up on my ass. It surprised me I made it through the day with no falls. Kyle came home early from work and convinced me to have one of those evil muscle relaxants that I hate to take. The same pills that likely contributed to my psychotic episode. I was receiving toxic doses when it happened, accompanied by a plethora of other medications.

We were supposed to attend the MS fall supper in Pincher Creek, but the weather was not prevailing so it was pushed to the end of October. Sadly, we had to miss the dinner. We would be back in Ottawa for my six month check-ups. I spent an hour on the phone crying to Ann over it. All of my sadness came from a selfish side of wanting to share our story. I say our story, because it is ours. Kyle, my family and I, it is all of ours to share equally. I want everyone to know there is hope for the future generations of our disease.

For my 40th birthday Kyle and I went for supper. It was fabulous way to start off a terrific night. My girlfriends picked me up at the restaurant and we headed over to my friend, Sherry's to get ready to go out. Another friend of mine, Mary, had gone shopping after she was finished work to find me a costume. While getting ready, out of the bag it came. It was a purple dress, I think it was a sexy wizard but

I'm not positive. I must say when my hair and makeup were done and I was dressed, I looked phenomenal. This was the best part of the rest of the evening out. Just to be with them. I climbed around twelve steep stairs. Kyle and I stayed in a hotel. It was easier to commute to the airport while in the city since our flight was the following day.

The next day Kyle and I packed and got ready for our flight. It was my first full day of walking unaided everywhere. I walked out of the hotel to the truck, and then at the park and jet I walked to the shuttle bus, then all through the Calgary airport. Standing is a big deal due to the fact that it uses all my muscle and strength and wears me down. What seemed to be the most uncomfortable was sitting on the plane for three hours. It is easy to get cramped up when you have nowhere to go.

When we finally arrived in Ottawa it was time to get off and get moving. Airport staff had brought me a chair thinking that I needed one. I got up, stretched out, and grabbed my walker, and headed up the walkway.

The following day was phenomenal! I was glad I stood my ground and didn't bring my wheelchair to my appointments. I knew, in my heart of hearts, I would be able to walk wherever I needed to go. I walked easily two miles around the hospital that day. All of my appointments went very well. They said that unless something went really sideways, they didn't need to see me out here again. This was wonderful news. Kyle and I went around that afternoon delivering pens our friend Jamie Lund of Sparwood made for us. We gave them as gifts to the people who saved my life.

It was bittersweet seeing all of the staff again, in 8 months I had developed many fond relationships.

The day after we arrived home we headed to the new South Campus Hospital in Calgary for an appointment with Dr. Pearson. She was so excited to see me and how well I was doing. So much in fact, she was near tears while we spoke. The last time she saw me was before my BMT, I was still in my wheelchair.

My new nurses at the MS Clinic were very nice, though they were not Kathy. Over the years I became very reliant on her because she was always a phone call away. Since my diagnosis, she had the ability to settle my fears, curb my tears or whatever other sense of dismay I may have gotten myself into.

Kyle and I decided to visit Kathy at the Foothills Hospital one day.

After our visit he said, "Fiona we should walk over to the 11th floor to show you off to the nurses up there."

My immediate reaction was, "no way in hell am I going up there." I was so ashamed of my behavior when I was a resident of the 11th floor, which is the Neurological Unit at the Foothills Hospital. It is where I stayed while having my lapse of sanity, before the psych ward. While I was stark raving mad I was scornfully mean to everyone.

It took some persuading but, Kyle was finally able to convince me to go upstairs. When we came around the corner to the nurse's station we saw the head clerk and I immediately felt better. She was smiling at us and this diminished my fear of the reunion. We requested to see old staff and once the astonishment passed; there were plenty of smiles, laughter and gratitude to go around. We were informed that some of the staff had transferred to different floors of the hospital so we went down a few floors. Downstairs we visited with staff that saw me at my absolute worst. There were even a few people who were keeping up with me through my blog the entire time we were in Ottawa. How special this made me feel. That they cared enough about me to follow my life brings grateful tears. Many thanks to Kyle for convincing me to go, it was a redeeming feeling.

I started experiencing bouts of pain in my ligaments. It was going to take some time getting used to these new symptoms. I had a hard time coping with this new pain. I tried desperately to grasp why it ensued after the transplant.

I ended another cycle of antibiotics. It seemed within hours I was symptomatic again. By this point it had been six months since the recurrent infection had started. Needless to say, I was quite fed up. God was looking out for me, testing my will and when I was ready to give up, he'd loosen the slack.

One morning after having my morning coffee with Kyle, I went for a shower. On the way to the shower I walked across the kitchen. The pace of my steps was quick and I was enthused.

"That was not the test," Kyle said as he came around the corner.

I spun around and smiled. I turned around and walked backwards down the hall. It was quite some time since I could independently walk backwards. I walked backwards ten steps without touching a wall or losing my balance. I kicked it up a notch. I balanced myself and stood on one foot. Kyle reached out his hands and my fingers feathered his. I stood on one foot and then the other.

November 11<sup>th</sup> finally rolled around and Kyle and I celebrated this precious anniversary. The day I was admitted to the Ottawa General Hospital to start the treatment for my procedure.

Come December, our family had their share of heartache with deaths within the family. It made Christmas feel off. I lost a cousin, an aunt and two uncles in the past year.

The beginning of December we received another call that my aunt would be passing soon, we were told she had three days. We lost five members from my Moms side of the family this year. It distressed my mother's heart.

There is an upside to sorrow. We had the chance to love them and plenty of memories to share. We didn't feel too cheated by their passing. They had lived meaningful and eventful lives, and we got to share that with them. I have been blessed and I am truly honored to have and have had such wonderful people in my life.

December is the anniversary month of my transplant and I decided to post old blog entries with my new ones. I did this so my readers and I could see the comparison, just how far I had come in a year. The difference was something beyond words.

I received an amazing machine to help with my circulation and muscle spasms. It's called the Revitive Circulation Booster. It is the most magical unit I have ever used, giving me the ability to stretch an extra four inches past my toes. I could put my hands on this cool machine and it somehow worked so I that I was able to close my fingers in the morning without feeling pain.

December 29, 2012 was my 1st birthday for my second chance at life. I know, you're probably wondering, how many birthdays does this woman have? But each one signifies pivotal moments within my life. All absolutely essential for me to become the person I am today, who is still here today. On December 29th, just one year prior I was an empty shell, my entire body had been wiped clean and I was waiting for my new cells to take hold.

Upon waking Christmas morning, I knew it was going to be great day. I was with my family, maybe not perfectly healthy, certainly by far better than I had been in the last three years. I spent this Christmas surrounded by everyone I love most, my parents, my sister and of course, my Kyle.

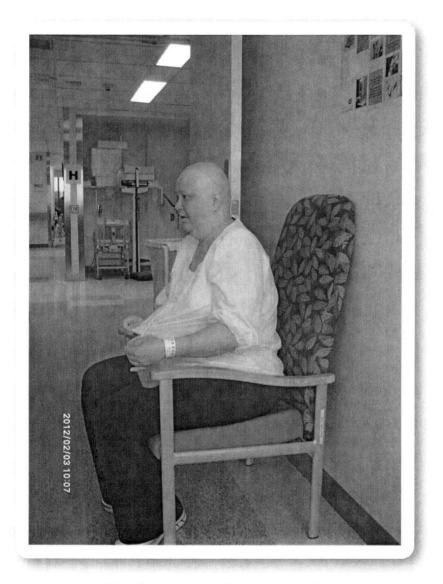

*First day wearing clothes in two months*

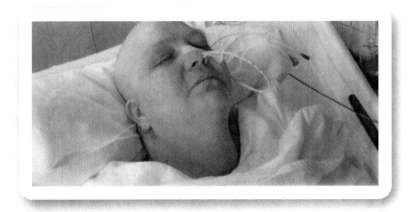

*Me and my feeding tube*

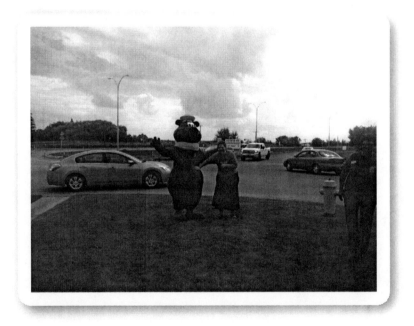

*Me and the A&W mascot bear raising money for MS*

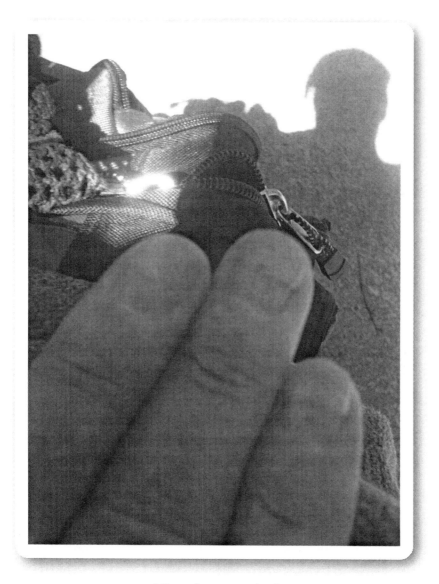

*My nails growing back*

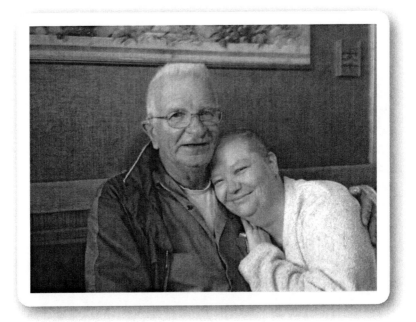

*Ralph and I at breakfast*

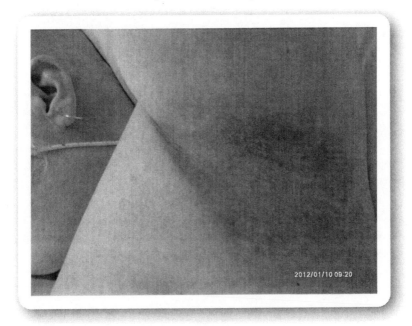

*The blood that pooled in my armpit*

# The Yo-Yo Effect

EARLY JANUARY 2013 MY UROLOGIST, DR. BAVERSTOCK, BOOKED me in for Botox injections on my bladder. My bladder spasms make me squirt urine. The Botox relaxes my bladder and stops the spasms.

Dr. Baverstock walked into the examination room with my file in his hand.

"Fiona, I am always happy when I see your name on my list. I never know if you're going to be alive for your next appointment. There have been too many changes over the years." He said with a smile on his face as he came around the corner of the curtain.

Getting ready for the Botox injections, nurses placed my feet into elevated stirrups, and then Dr. Baverstock stuck twenty needles into my bladder. Yes, it is as painful as it sounds. They did freeze me beforehand, but they stick in the needles almost immediately after, so the freezing doesn't make much of a difference.

It reminds me of when Doctor Freedman stuck a needle in the

back of my skull to deaden a nerve that was causing extreme pain in my ear. The bladder injections aren't as painful as the needle in my head, but it does stir up memories.

I had the Botox procedure done 5 times prior to my transplant. I would end up with an infection that landed me in the hospital every time. This procedure, post-transplant, was the first time the Botox did not cause temporary paralysis. This is an example of one of the many reasons I have gratitude for the transplant. It's changed my life in so many profound ways.

I found out Alberta Aides to Daily Living (AADL) would only cover 70 catheters every two months. This would be fine if I didn't have to catheterize 6 times a day. Each package specifically states that they are for one use only. I was directed to rewash and reuse. This is kind of predicament for someone who suffers from consistent UTI and bladder infections. Even with minimal benefits I received, it is hard to imagine what I will do when my long term disability expires in three years.

I learned many lessons adapting to my post-transplant body. One of my lessons learned is when I forget to take my nightly "pee pill" called Desmopressin. I would wake up with an overflowing diaper and a soaked bed.

I stopped taking a medication called Valtrex that I had been given to combat side effects from my treatments. The moment I stopped, the inside of my mouth was covered in cold sores.

I contracted shingles and it was the roughest feeling I have experienced since arriving home from Ottawa. My body reacted to the virus making my legs wobbly and I could barely stand.

I had chills and awful spasms. While sitting on the sofa, I felt something and it scared me quite a bit. I hadn't felt this since I was a paraplegic. I felt like I was being torn in half from the ridge that runs right below my breasts. The feeling only lasted a short period of time, but it made me discover my fears of becoming sicker were still prominent.

I met a new friend named Karen who is also battling MS. It was nice to finally speak to someone who has similarities in the severity of our disease. Another battle in common, she also had the transplant.

I have quite a few friends who suffer from MS; I guess you could say birds of a feather flock together. I think it is crucial for people suffering from our disease to have empathetic support. It makes all the difference when you can talk to someone walking in similar shoes.

Nonetheless my health improved, regardless of my symptomatic setbacks. One particular day stands out to me. I will share it with you so you can have an understanding of what an exceptionally good and productive day for me can consist of.

One morning I awoke with a zest for life that I seemingly had not felt in many years. I crawled out of bed and jumped in the shower. It felt wonderful to take my first shower in weeks without requiring a chair. To stand upright unaided, with the lovely feeling of water running over your body is something most take for granted. If you didn't before, perhaps you can appreciate it now. Itchy was lying peacefully on my bed sleeping until I was out, dried and dressed. It was a remarkable start to my day to accomplish all of this before 8:30 am.

We went to town and when Itchy and I arrived home I put her in the back yard. I took a much needed rest on the couch for an hour or so, and then I emailed information to my work. Sitting down too long causes me to seize up so when that happens I get up and find something else to do. I played music and cleaned my kitchen, a good thorough clean that included moving objects and mopping. I two stepped around the kitchen while completing these tasks, having a great time. For an MS patient, just the mobility aspect of this day makes it spectacular.

When Kyle arrived home I playfully turned the music on again. I tried to show him my moves from earlier in the day but I lost my balance and fell into our solid oak table. He wasn't impressed. I gave my ribs and back quite an ass kicking because twenty minutes after the fall my breathing felt painful.

Kyle gets upset with me for good reasons. It is not so much my silly behavior while he's home that is worrisome, but what I do when he is not around. I could be grateful that such falls no longer resulted in a hospital visit, before my transplant, every fall lead to a hospitalization. I've had several falls since Ottawa and not one hospitalized me.

Another day, my spirit was soaring. I left home early in the morning and had time to spare all day. On my way through the Pass I had time to stop and photograph the mountains. I gave the truck a wash, happy to have the strength to do it.

On my way home I had called Kyle to let him know I would be arriving soon.

He asked where I was and I responded while cackling, "In the truck!"

"Where in the truck?" He asked, I laughed even harder.

"Behind the steering wheel," I chirped smugly.

"Okay you smart ass, where is the truck?"

I roared, "On the highway!" I laughed so hard I almost had to pull over.

These days are examples of when I was blessed to feel 'normal' again. I had my independence back, if only for a moment. I know that eventually it will be gone, seemingly as quickly as I had grasped it. But I can always look forward to its return. That notion, by itself is a blessing to consider.

I started conforming to all the positive aspects of my life. It gave me a new understanding of why things are the way they are. Why I was the way I was and why I am the way I am now. There was clarity brewing beneath the surface of my existence, waiting for me to discover it with honesty and gratitude.

I had an enlightening conversation with Karen and my mother. I was approaching nearly 22 years of sobriety and reflecting on my recovery. I had an epiphany with my relationship with denial. As an alcoholic, denial could have killed me. When it came to my disease, it was denial that saved me. Denial had kept me going long enough for the procedure. Before the procedure I chose not to believe what the doctors were telling me. I honestly did not clue into the fact that I was as sick as I was until Dr. Freedman stated so at our first meeting. I learned early on that acceptance is the answer to all my problems today. My epiphany was that if I had accepted my fate when I was told to, I would not be here today.

I shared my epiphany with my mother and she said, "Dad and I would be visiting you at the Kevisville Cemetery." Acceptance is crucial, but everything happens for a reason.

I had another epiphany that was profound. I felt guilty for being given the gift of a second chance when there are so many people in my life who deserve it too. I was lost between two different worlds. When I was dying I did not fit with the 'normal' MS patients. I was so sick that I felt like I had a completely different disease. Then, after my transplant and some recovery, I felt the same dissimilarity. This time it was from the other side of the fence, I was getting better and stronger every day. The people who looked at me with pity before now looked at me with envy.

My friend Denise said, "It sounds kind of like survivors guilt." That's exactly what it was.

Near the end of March I received an email from Global News medical reporter. I was beside myself with excitement. My story was going to get some media attention. This was an excellent way to share the miracle of the procedure I received. Karen would come from Victoria, BC to stay with me and partake in the interview with Global News.

On March 26, 2013 Kyle and I picked Karen up from the airport.

On March 27th Karen accompanied me to the gym while I worked out. I ended up doing a second workout because the news crew wanted footage.

After the gym we headed to my house to do the interviews. It was a big deal for me. There was a lot of excitement surrounding my fifteen minutes of fame.

Afterwards, Karen attended Easter dinner with my family. It was a lovely evening and I was happy she was able to meet my family and share a holiday meal with us. On April 1st we brought Karen back to the airport for an emotional farewell.

I saw Dr. Pearson and she was so impressed with my recovery she was at a loss for words. I never guessed in our six year relationship she was capable of being speechless. She performed all the standard neurological testing, stunned by how well I was doing. She told me that I, out of all her other patients, had made the most progress. She said she had never seen anyone make such an extensive transformation in her career. It was one hell of a compliment to Dr. Freedman, Dr. Atkins and I. They fought so very hard to save not just my life, but the lives of many others.

For the first time since my diagnosis 8 years ago, I only had to see my neurologist once a year. I have NEVER been well enough for that.

It was bittersweet and I felt a little lost. I'd been surrounded by medical staff for so long that, not seeing them for a year was beyond my comprehension. It was outstanding, but the change would require some adjustment.

The following months I crossed milestone after milestone. I couldn't be stopped. I shopped by myself, using a basket and not relying on a cart to lean on. At one point I held a basket with two mini watermelons, a bunch of bananas and a bag of oranges, all while holding my purse on the other side of my shoulder.

There was a time when I could not carry a purse because it would throw my balance off and likely lead to a fall.

I walked a mile and a half twice a week and strength trained three times a week.

I mentioned before how I had a great fear of boarding elevators, you can imagine how out of the question escalators were. I wouldn't even dare before. I conquered that fear and I rode an escalator for the first time since being diagnosed!

While enjoying my freedom, poor sweet Kyle had to adjust to these changes as well. He never knew me healthy. I was always an injured little bird. He went from knowing every single detail of my daily routine to not knowing if I was home or not. Of course he was concerned; at times even I had a hard time grasping how healthy I was.

My relationship with Teena improved as well. In April 2013, I revealed my deep, dark secret of my rape to her. Ironically, our relationship has flourished ever since. On mother's day I revealed my secret to my mother.

Once my sister and my mother knew, I felt free to write anything. I had shared the secret in meetings and with my sponsor, but this wasn't enough.

In example, if one of my girls had been raped, I would by help them sharing my experience with them, encouraging them to talk about their experiences. So they could know they weren't alone. Until writing this book, I had not fully dealt with my rape because I still had never told my family. There was still a lot of shame. Once my mother and sister knew I was released from the burden of shame because they didn't look at me any differently. They still accepted me.

On June 15th a memorial service was held for dearest Ralph. Two years had passed since his initial disappearance. His family felt it was time to start grieving the loss of our beloved Ralph. I was asked by his family to do Ralph's eulogy. I can't remember a time in my life where I have felt this level of love and gratitude. While gathering information to write the eulogy I learned more about Ralph in the weeks leading up to the memorial than I had known in the 20+ years we were friends. Ralph was my best friend, always my go-to fella. He was the kind of person who was always there for everyone else. He taught me many things while accompanying me on trips in my big truck. He was a fountain of knowledge. The loss I felt that day cut me deeper than anything I have felt in a very long time. Years ago my mother was concerned that Ralph and I were too close. She feared that if he passed away I would turn to drinking again. Keep in mind this was an earlier time, while I was still young in the program. Ralph was the same age as my parents, but it felt like we were two peas, maybe not sharing a pod, but certainly from the same patch of garden.

On the day of his memorial I was heartbroken. I felt the pain of the deep and hollow hole there was going to be in my life. He was not coming back. To this day I think of him daily. I was truly honored that his family asked me to speak at his service and say farewell. I'm eternally grateful for his presence in my life. He was a force to be reckoned with, he had a spirit of an angel and I will miss him forever.

On June 25, 2013 we flew back to Ottawa for follow up appointments. We checked back into that familiar Rotel. The next day we made our rounds, running into familiar faces and hospital staff.

When I saw Dr. Atkins he was astonished with my progress. He looked over the results of the transplant and he used the word, "miracle" more than once. In the middle of the meeting I had to use the bathroom and Dr. Atkins watched me closely as I stood out of my chair, strolled out of the room and down the hall.

He was absolutely stunned.

When I returned he said, "If I have never before seen a miracle, I just did."

This statement coming from a scientist meant the world to me.

My next appointment was with Dr. Freedman. He measured me on The Kurtzke Expanded Disability Status Scale (EDSS) which is a method of quantifying disability in MS. The same scale I had to pass to receive the procedure. It's a scale measuring from 1 to 10 in half point increments, ten being labeled as "death due to MS". I was measuring at a 3.5, the best score I have received since my diagnosis. Throughout my illness I averaged a 6 to 6.5. At my worst in 2011 I was a 9.0 which is, "helpless bed patient; can communicate and eat".

It was celebratory news. Kyle and I were happy we were making better memories in Ottawa. We visited with our friends we had made there and left feeling a little heartsick, but mostly content.

When I got home I sifted through more paperwork. I've come to the conclusion that I was one lucky lady to have Alberta healthcare. The first three years after my diagnosis I was being covered for $5000 medications each month, granted it was more expensive because of my inability to go into remission. Back then a patient had to pay for their own shots if they didn't have a certain amount of relapses. Once again, it is another situation where the severity of my illness ended up helping me out with the circumstances. For the first year and a half I was on [30]Copaxone. It had barely had an affect so they put me on [31]Rebif for another year and a half. Going into my fourth and fifth years I received chemotherapy once a month for over a year and then it stopped working. I had two sessions of Plasmapheresis for ten days. They used six bottles each day of the ten days and the serum is VERY expensive. They do this treatment on many different people with multitudes of diseases and it is all covered by the Alberta government. I feel blessed to be Canadian.

In July I was diagnosed with hyperthyroidism. Not long after I had my port catheter removed. I had this catheter since 2010. Having the port removed was another step closer to being free of my past. That little contraption had meant the world to me while it was in. It meant even more now that it was out. It was the last piece of equipment in my body from the last three years. I've had two different main lines in my neck, a dual PICC-line in my arm and finally, my port. After

---

30   Copaxone is a synthetic protein made up of a combination of four amino acids that chemically resemble a component of myelin (the insulating material that protects nerves and helps them work properly). Copaxone induces the production of immune cells that are less damaging to myelin. Source: http://mssociety.ca/en/treatments/modify_copaxone.htm

31   Rebif is a beta-interferon that is produced from mammalian cells using recombinant DNA techniques (a series of procedures used to join together DNA segments). Beta-interferon is a protein that occurs naturally in the human body in response to initiating factors such as viruses. In MS, the main effects of Rebif are to block the activity of certain immune system cells and to reduce the passage of these immune cells into the central nervous system, where they cause inflammation and damage to myelin (the insulating material that protects nerves and helps them work properly). Source: http://mssociety.ca/en/treatments/modify_rebif.htm

it was removed they let me keep it and it felt odd staring at it as it sat on the coffee table. With three stitches in my chest where the port used to be, it really felt like this was the end of the road for all of the hardships I had endured in the last eight years.

I felt now, more prominently than ever, this was the start of a new life. I had to have a purpose, God had other plans for me or none of this would have come to pass.

I had to be revaccinated for all the shots that infants receive after being born. The doctors were feeling confident and weaning back my medication to see how I would fare. I tried to stop taking a medication that helped with my walking. Dr. Freedman wanted to see if I still needed it, but a few days later I was already experiencing balance issues and put back on my medication, Frampyra.

August was an eventful month for me. I attended my father's 72$^{nd}$ birthday and celebrated my 22$^{nd}$ sober birthday. Teena and I planned a party and celebrated my parent's 50$^{th}$ anniversary. I spent a month going through pictures to show on a big screen. We sent out formal invitations, it was just like planning the wedding all over with a decorated head table and all. The party was huge success. We had a head count of nearly 200 people, a full house. We were so grateful everyone came. Near the end of August I won the 2013 Donna Thurber Courage Award, what an honor to be recognized in that fashion.

My thyroid was becoming quite troublesome, I lost thirty five pounds since coming home from Ottawa and the hot flashes were horrific. I was an emotional rollercoaster and more weepy than usual for it. My thyroid was producing double the hormone needed so they treated me with radiated iodine. They would let the iodine accumulate in the thyroid gland and it would kill a portion of it. This would result in it producing less of the hormone; thereafter I would take a supplement to regulate my numbers. My overactive thyroid didn't just affect my mood or my body temperature. It felt like it was triggering MS symptoms. Any sort of imbalance within my body caused a flare up with my MS, what a bothersome characteristic for this disease. As always, Kyle, my knight in shining armour always came to my rescue during these awful times.

September proved my cognitive functions were returning so I decided to get my GED. I succeeded in my courses and aced my lesson exams. The only way to keep improving was to continue picking up the pieces and move on.

The start of October 2013 was a pain in the ass. My thyroid went from hyper to hypo. I gained 15 pounds in 3 days. Back to the endocrinologist I went. October 26th I turned 41. This is the second birthday I wouldn't have had if not for the stem cell transplant. I couldn't help but think, well here I am dammit! Everything is amazing, life is fabulous. My spectacular birthday started off with morning coffee with Kyle. After coffee, I attended a Saturday morning meeting. At the meeting I spoke of how I am grateful for every day because these are days I almost didn't have.

November was a better month. I started sleeping on my side. I haven't slept on my side since 2006 when I started wearing diapers. Sleeping on my side was impossible as incontinence diapers have no protection on the sides. Sleeping on my back was the only safe way to sleep. An excellent reminder of how far I have come. I made an informational video on YouTube about bladder Botox and the Ottawa MS Society used it for their website.

November 18th Kyle was scheduled for surgery, a [32]Stapedectomy which is a surgical procedure of the middle ear performed to improve hearing. I sat waiting for him while he was in surgery all afternoon. He went in at 2 pm and into recovery at 5. I hadn't been on this side of health fence in a very long time. As a child I spent many hours that felt like days in hospital waiting rooms. This day gave me some insight how everyone must have felt time after time. Countless hours of waiting for news, praying for the best. Now, sitting here waiting for Kyle I had no clue how he had such a calm demeanour all those months. He truly is an amazing man.

November 28th I attended a going away party for Ann who was moving to Arizona. The event was in a ballroom and I walked up the grand staircase to enter it. Then I sang and danced. I DANCED. It was like seeing a close friend after too much time passed, and I only lost my balance a couple times. After the dance I walked down the

---

32    Source: http://en.wikipedia.org/wiki/Stapedectomy

grand staircase. The entire night was absolutely astonishing. It was a sensational farewell and tribute to the woman who launched me towards my wellbeing.

I didn't find out until the 1st of December, but the same night as Ann's farewell ceremony a dear friend of mine was killed in a car accident on his way home from work. He was killed by a drunk driver. I won't mention his name out of respect for his grieving family. This man was a huge part of helping me get through my resentments from my accident with the drunk driver. He was killed at 33 years sober. When I was hit I was 13 years sober. Now all I can do is give to others what he has given me over the decades. He was the friend that helped me see that the tables could have been turned. When I was drinking it could have been me that hit and hurt someone else. My love and prayers go out to all his friends and family, it is still a devastating loss.

A few days later Kyle and I ran into one of my old nurses in the Pass. This nurse had not seen me since I had been sent home to die. She was excited to hear I was in remission. I have all the damage incurred prior to the transplant which is why I am sporadically symptomatic. But I'm alive. Seeing people now, after being so ill – their reactions really validate my progress.

Christmas was blissfully normal. Everything went off without a fuss. I got to assist my parents instead of vice versa and that was an enjoyable feeling. Filled with gratitude and reflection, I enjoyed another holiday I might have missed out on if not for the procedure. We were all merrier for it.

December 29, 2013 was my 2<sup>nd</sup> post-transplant birthday. Many

things had changed for me over the last year and a half of freedom.

I felt release from the bondage of a disease that was not so slowly

killing me. A disease that continues to do this to many people I love

and hundreds of thousands more. I wish everyone suffering can

have the freedom that I've been given. I welcomed 2014, knowing

it would start the furthest I have ever been from this disease since

being diagnosed.

*2014*

2014 started off just as 2013 ended. My body continued to progress in

the same fashion until March.

Everything kicked up a notch in March.

March 1<sup>st</sup> felt like a whirlwind of positivity. Kyle and I awakened

like any other weekend and at 10 o'clock am, the phone rang. Our

friends called, asking if they could view the house. I was grateful that

Kyle and I had meticulously gone over the house the week before for

a viewing that ended up being cancelled.

He tried to settle me as I dusted like a mad woman, "they've been

here many times, the viewing is only a formality." I couldn't stop.

During the viewing, the moment our friend's wife began measuring to see if their dining room table would fit, I knew they would be taking it. Kyle laughed at me when I told him this after they left.

I said, "I don't know much, but I know how women think."

The following six weeks were quite stressful. We only had six weeks to find a new home and we ended up lucking out. We found another house on an acreage near Trochu that suited us perfectly. By now, you are aware of the consequences from stress and what it inflicts on a MS patient. I had to take some off days during this time, battling horrific muscle spasms and crippling fatigue. Between packing, paperwork and everything changing, I was exhausted.

We moved into our dream home in Trochu, AB on April 12th. Overjoyed my body was cooperating, Kyle and I busily prepared the house and yard. It gave me a nostalgic reminder of when I was back on the farm. I pruned away saplings, I was up and down and crawling all around. I even unpacked the kitchen. While doing all of this, I suffered spasms and fatigue in the evening, symptoms that were worth enduring to be on our beautiful acreage.

Shortly after we moved in I found out that the Lido Café, a restaurant Ralph and I had frequented, was shut down. The loss of the restaurant made me feel like I had lost another piece of Ralph. We had spent hours sitting at the tables in the Lido, sharing our lives. I sat crying in my new home, realizing that this is the first place I moved into in the last 23 years that Ralph has never physically been in. He would have loved it here.

It is also the only place that I didn't have a spare room for him. Everywhere I have ever lived since meeting Ralph I have always had a spare room for him.

Who would think that a restaurant closing its doors would be so clarifying? Ralph had been a constant figure in my life for so long that it didn't seem real that he was gone until the Lido shut its doors. I remember speaking with my mom about how long it would take before his loss became real. I'm very grateful that he guided me through grievances while he was still here. He taught me to grieve in a healthy way. Even with him gone, he continued to teach me.

Sadly, by May I was not as well as I had been. It seemed the cause was from stress of the move. Kyle and my loved ones asked me to slow down, but I didn't want to. The first week in June I lost my balance in the kitchen and fell down.

June was the beginning of a terrifying period for me and all of those who love me. The entire months of June and July I used my walker fulltime.

By July 21$^{st}$ my family doctor advised me to try Prednisone. A week later I saw my neuro-ophthalmologist, Dr. Costello and she gave me the same advice. I wasn't happy with the direction this was headed in. Only a few days later my MS nurse called wanting me to start a high dose of steroids. I was not in favor of this. It was a scary thought to think the Prednisone might work. It meant I would be in relapse. This shouldn't be possible, the procedure was supposed to halt my disease.

I wasn't pleased with the thought of blowing up like a balloon either. Steroids always made me retain so much fluid. I felt disappointed I would have to go through this treatment again. I had an appointment with my MS nurse on the 29th, at this appointment we would know if I was relapsing. I knew I would be able to tell within a few days.

My doctor booked me for an MRI on August 23rd. I asked the universe to make it so the steroids had no effect. I hoped my body was simply mad with me for overdoing it.

I was directed to take 1250 mg of prednisone every 2nd day for 10 days. The dosage was so high I barely slept and my body felt bizarre. A feeling I am more familiar with than I care to admit. Within a couple of doses I started to swell and my clothes didn't fit. My skin was tender, the swelling made it impossible to wear a bra because I felt bruised. I couldn't believe I was here again. I talked to Marjorie in Ottawa; she wasn't very pleased I was back on steroids.

Kyle grew angry and it broke my heart. He wasn't angry with me. He was frustrated with my symptoms. Looking into his eyes I saw that the anger was fear based.

The reality was frightening for both of us.

"What will be, will be." Kyle would say.

"It is what it is," my mother commented.

We were back on Fiona's merry-go-round. No sense in getting worked up over what we can't control.

Marjorie encouraged me to keep busy and I was grateful to hear this. Everyone else had been telling me to do nothing, to sit, relax and let my body heal. Marjorie and I were on the same page. No movement for me is just as detrimental as too much.

One particular day I accomplished a lot and I couldn't help but think of my dear friend Ralph and how he used to say, "Make a plan, not a prediction." How I wish he were here now to offer me his words of wisdom. His absence often crept up on me, making my heart ache.

My first week on Prednisone made me feel better, but in a conflicting way. What Prednisone does for me and what it does to me are two very different effects. Prednisone gives me the opportunity to partake in life again, as well as the ability to take care of myself and those I love. On the other hand, the side effects are unpleasant. I lose sleep for days at a time and I swell up until I'm the size of a water buffalo.

On July 29$^{th}$ I took my final high dose. Starting the next day I would begin a weaning period, on a smaller dose continued for 10 more days.

One day when I had to pee an old and familiar tribulation occurred. I desperately tried to hold it long enough to make it inside the store from my vehicle.

I parked and when I stood up my bladder released.

I continued into the store and went straight into the bathroom. I put my pants in the sink and washed them, rinsed them and wrung them out. Then I redressed.

Memories flooded my mind during this process. I had stood at too many sinks, for too many years cleaning soiled clothing. Here I was again, repeating the wretched cycle. I drove around the rest of the day with a sweater on my seat.

I left the house in my wheelchair on August 9th and it was the first time in 3 years I required it. Reality was painstakingly sinking in and I realized the days ahead were uncertain.

I had to use my shower chair again. I would wait for Kyle to come home from work before I could shower because I required his assistance entering and exiting the tub. This moment was the most difficult for my heart to accept.

I had recently joined the Lions Club. There were roughly 10 stairs to climb when entering the building. I wore my moccasins so I was able to slide my feet and shuffle easier. To get up the stairs, Kyle walked my right leg while I pulled up my left behind me. More familiar trials. Everything was hard to acknowledge. I felt angry, scared, lost and confused.

Questions flooded my mind when I woke in the morning. Would I be able to move today? Where do I go from here? Do I still have a future? Am I strong enough to take it?

Am I dying?

I felt heaviness in my torso and my limbs and they continued feeling heavier. Kyle would lay me down before he went to sleep on days I couldn't get into bed on my own. He was certainly more optimistic than I felt.

"We will just look at you tomorrow and see what happens," he would say lovingly. He took a wonderful approach to my circumstances. Moments like this I am reminded that this is not just my life anymore. It is ours.

August 14, 2014 was the day after my last dose of prednisone. This day brought on some clarity and acceptance for me. I was not giving up on getting better, but I needed to accept what was happening to me. I knew that if I did not accept my fate I would be consumed by unhappiness and bitterness. These feelings aren't very productive, especially if your time is limited. My body was rapidly failing 40 hours after finishing my last dose. I could no longer ignore the symptoms or pray they would get better.

While speaking with Teena one day she looked at a picture of me from when I had lost all my hair in Ottawa. She said that hair is nothing more than accessory. I began to realize that my body, too, is merely an accessory. I decided that as long as my mind, heart and spirit were clear and free, I could live with that. My body didn't impact who I was, it simply held my soul.

I had to accept that I was now back in a place I never thought I would return to again. With Kyle working I required assistance during the day. I grudgingly made arrangements to have Home Care come and assist me while Kyle was at work. My condition was so poor I was set up in no time with daily aides. They cut up my food and washed my undercarriage. An occupational therapist was setting up the house to meet my needs. A physiotherapist came twice a week, helping me maintain my strength. Kyle was building a wheelchair ramp when he wasn't working. He was bustling to get it complete before the snow came. There was so much going on and I was a hostage in my own home. Being confined to my chair, I was trapped in the house until the ramp was completed. I was terrified, consumed that I was in full relapse.

My body steadily declined with no explanation. By September 1st my fatigue became unbearable. I got up in the middle of the night to use the washroom and nodded off as I sat on the toilet. I'm not sure if I came woke as I fell off the toilet or when I hit the floor but, by the time I was fully aware, my raised toilet seat was lying on top of me.

In the morning I called Life Line and they set up their services almost immediately.

Not too long after this I required an indwelling catheter; it was getting too difficult and dangerous to transfer me to the toilet. Things were definitely going downhill, at a faster pace than ever before.

I had a couple of visits with the Chaplin's at the South Campus Hospital in Calgary. Kyle had been with me for the 2nd visit. We discussed whether I was okay with dying and I was. I asked them if they believed me, if they thought I was really accepting of my fate, or just in denial. I felt grateful when they both responded that they felt my acceptance was soul deep.

I started another cycle of Prednisone in September that lasted until October. I ended my final regime the day before Thanksgiving. We had Thanksgiving at my house this year. My family was extremely nervous, no one knew what to expect from me on my first day without the steroids. Luckily, I was okay, just tired. Kyle was the savior of Thanksgiving. He did all the cooking, setting and serving. My sister gave me a beautiful butterfly necklace because she believed I might not make it to see Christmas. This is a good example of the reality we were living with.

My spasms became crippling and the dosage for my muscle relaxants, Tizanidine and Baclofen were increased. I was able to wean down a bit by November 2014.

November 19th my homecare aid came at 1 pm to get me ready for the day. The aid clamped my catheter hose to clean my bag, which was part of the bag cleansing ritual. After we finished, she left and I got on with my day. I didn't realize anything was wrong until around 9 that evening. It was bed time and I was feeling very uncomfortable.

I said to Kyle, "I have to go get these pants off." I couldn't understand why I was so uncomfortable.

Then I went to drain my bag and discovered it was empty.

I felt a wave of panic and then I remembered the clamp. Holy crap the clamp!

I removed the clamp and my bag filled with 1150 milliliters of urine. A bladder shouldn't hold more than 800, most empty at around 600.

Sadly, this particular aid had done the same thing a couple of weeks earlier but I realized the error within 4 hours. This mistake blew my unknown sub-clinical UTI into a full blown UTI.

The next day on November 22$^{nd}$ I woke screaming in agony at 2 am. I recognized this discomfort; my catheter line was blocked again. I reached down to feel for the clamp on my line but could find none. I knew I was in big trouble. I pulled at the line to see if I could dislodge whatever was impeding the flow but I couldn't. Terrified and desperate, I called Kyle who woke up and rushed to my room. When he could not help me he called 911. Thankfully, there was no need to be transported to the hospital. The paramedics were able to clear the blockage in my line with a syringe of water.

On November 23$^{rd}$ things took a turn for the worse.

After waking Kyle helped me into my chair. I drained my catheter bag and when I turned out of the bathroom I felt a horrible pain in my left shoulder blade. Moments later, the same pain in my left hip. By this point my entire left side was paralyzed. I struggled to get myself to the kitchen where Kyle was. He looked at me and immediately knew that something was very wrong. He performed a stroke test and I passed. I rolled into the living room and sat by the fire. I remember thinking it was odd that Kyle had checked my neck to see if it would turn, this was something no one had ever done before. As I sat in the living room, I realized that the rest of my body was paralyzed. I tried to turn my head and couldn't at all. I called out to Kyle, telling him to dial 911.

It was a good thing my O.T. had put a lift in my house because it assisted the paramedics while transferring me from my chair top the stretcher. I was taken to the hospital by ambulance; it had been over 2.5 years since my last stay.

The first day and half I was unable to move anything. When people spoke to me I would ask them to turn my head so I could face them. I felt like a marionette.

I wondered if the aid had not been so poor at her job that day, if I would have continued to go downhill without explanation. The doctors at the hospital put me on the correct antibiotic for my UTI, and once again, another 3 days of Intravenous Prednisone. The upside to all that was happening is that I was recovering. I wasn't relapsing, I was recovering. All of these terrible symptoms that lead me to home care and life line were from a sub-clinical UTI. Now I knew what to pay attention to.

With the correct antibiotic and Prednisone it wasn't long before I was walking unaided again. Putting myself to bed, cleaning, exercising, living my life, and grateful for every moment of it.

The reason why my UTI had been sub-clinical for so long was likely due to my prescription for Macrobid. An antibiotic I used as a prophylactic for many years as a means to hold off bladder infections. I learned at the end of this very long and grueling nine months that it was likely I had a subclinical UTI the entire time.

I thank God every day that I am optimistic by nature. It makes it easier to get through all the trying times. Because I had walked the same path of possible demise, I already had an idea of how to accept my fate. Truthfully, it really did seem easier to accept death the second time around. The most difficult aspect of everything was watching the sadness that engulfed Kyle and my family. There is no greater pain felt than that of watching your loved ones suffer. Then again, there is nothing more joyous than seeing their smiles of joy and relief upon learning I would be okay.

One early morning in December 2014 Kyle woke me at 2:30 am. He came in my room when the sky was clear of clouds. We went onto our back deck and sat in comfortable chairs Kyle had put towels on to keep our bums dry and warm. The stars were like diamonds glistening in the sky. The air was cool, snow blanketed over our yard, making it look like a blank canvas. I was dressed in my pajamas, wool sweater and winter boots. Kyle brought a blanket to protect me from the wind. The telescope was still packed away but we had the binoculars. It wasn't needed on this night anyway, the sky was clear. This is the first time since we moved here that we've taken the time to enjoy the beauty of the night sky together. This realization brings me to tears. We had been so consumed with the move and my getting sick again. It didn't matter now though, because I am back and my health is steadily returning. Kyle is at peace, and we took the time to watch the stars. I am grateful.

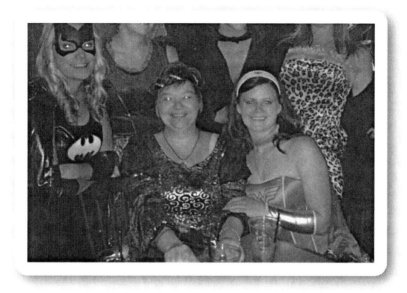

*Mary, me and Adrian out for my birthday on Halloween*

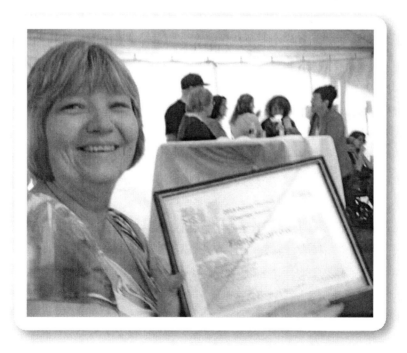

*Me with my Donna Thurber Courage Award*

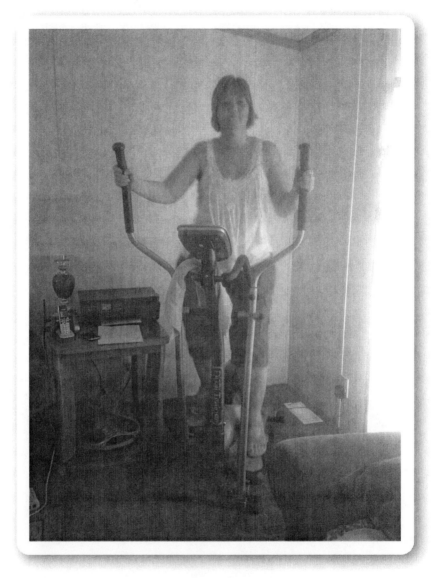

*Me exercising on the elliptical*

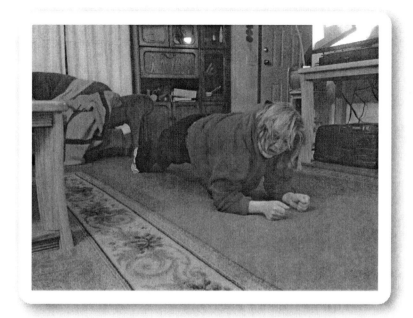

*Planking*

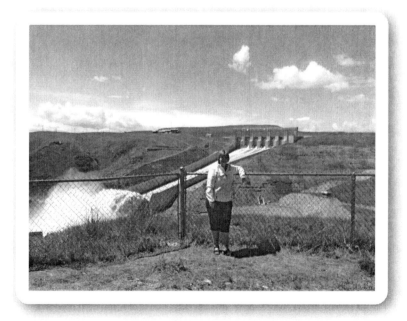

*The day I walked with both hands in my pockets for the first time*

# Final Word

TODAY MY LIFE IS SPECTACULAR. I'M HAPPY, JOYOUS AND FREE. Kyle and I are happy, well most of the time. I'm blessed to love and to be loved. I'm honored that I can share my story with you. I hope that my story can inspire courage and positivity within your own life, or at the very least, entertain you for a while.

I know I will never be able to give back all that I have received. I'm hoping my efforts and gratitude will suffice.

Four years ago I never would have predicted I would be where I am today. Four years ago I was in hospital, a terminal quadriplegic and fighting for my life.

This morning I exercised 30 minutes on my elliptical. Yesterday I was spring cleaning. I washed all my windows and many of my walls. Currently I am anticipating warm weather so I can take my dogs for a walk. The joy that having these abilities brings me is greater than I can explain. I am finally able to reciprocate the love and attention that was so tenderly bestowed upon me. I still have bad days, but I can always look forward to good ones returning.

While writing this book a couple things came to the forefront of my mind.

First is the painful secret I kept from my family for most of my life. I didn't realize how unresolved my feelings were until I tried to share it with you. In order to continue writing the book I had to confront my shame and confide in my sister and mother. After revealing my secret it gave me the freedom to put pen to paper.

Secondly, are the many losses I experienced due to my disease. Loss is a feeling I never really allowed myself to dwell in. I always fought past it, knowing that hanging onto that emotion was counterproductive. My life is only as good as I make it.

While writing this book I was faced with all of the losses I had endured. I relived each one, dwelled so that I could properly relay them to you.

The loss of my health and independence triggered by the fateful accident is the most prominent loss for me. Losing my ability to cross the border brought great angst and my career never felt the same. When it came to the loss of my career, I took it particularly hard. It took me some time to accept that I was done working. I lost my trucking buddy Moh and this still brings tears to my eyes. My failed relationship with Craig, 5 years lost. We were happy until my disease got the best of me, or at least I believed we were.

The loss of my freedom is my greatest sorrow, I feel it every day.

Some days when I remember how I thought my life would turn out, before getting sick. I am consumed with self-pity and grief. Then I look at all I have. Without these losses I wouldn't have the sense of gratitude I do. I wouldn't have the profound appreciation for life and all the blessings it has to offer.

The truth is, not every day will be good. Some days are still damned difficult. But I have a choice, I choose my reaction. I will continue to battle with the wreckage my disease left inside of my body. Some days the damage is blatantly apparent while other days it conceals itself fairly well. It is something I have to live with. But I am alive.

I am grateful for every great day I have, even the crap days. I am grateful for the added time I have been given. It makes every moment of every day more insightful. I have been given a second, a third and probably a fourth chance to live this life.

When I became ill again in 2014 I was reminded of how fast things can change. Maybe I needed this reminder. I spent hours on the phone with my mother, discussing what was really important in this life. During these conversations is when the awakenings of my true gratitude came to light. I had been given two and a half great years to love everyone. Time to heal old wounds that I didn't know I even had. Time to meet new friends, nurture the old ones and lose some that shouldn't have been there. It really is amazing how much can change, how much you can learn when simply given the time.

I thank God every day for giving me my trials when I had the strength to deal with them, even if I didn't have faith at the time. I am grateful my parents raised me right, this is why I had the clarity to sober up so young. They raised me to know right from wrong.

I am grateful for the 12 step program. Without the program I wouldn't have found my faith. My faith is the reason I am still here today. With my sobriety I gained knowledge of a higher power. I thank God for the right to question my faith. I look over my life today and know that there has always been a plan in place for my life.

I've questioned the higher power a lot throughout my life.

My dear friend Ralph asked me one day, "Fiona, when you close your eyes at night do you have the power to know if you are going to wake up?"

I said, "no, of course not."

"Then I am guessing there is something beyond our power. Whether you believe or not," he smiled.

From that moment I knew that whatever was in store for me, I would accept it and thrive in awareness. Throughout my years in program I have been taught that nothing, absolutely nothing happens in this world by mistake. It is with this knowledge that I am able to go forth optimistically one day at a time. There is uncertainty, but I know my higher power is holding my hand.

Having Multiple Sclerosis takes everything out of me some days. Days when I am standing at the stove making supper, the muscles in my legs become so weak that I collapse to the floor. Days when I am unable to wipe my own bottom because it causes muscle spasms up my back so terribly I seize up. Moments when I take a breath and cannot catch one. The moments when I try to swallow but I choke instead. It is the days when I attempt to take a step and, no matter how I try, I cannot. Nights I wish I could roll onto my side, but can't so I lay with tears of frustration rolling down my cheeks instead. Times I am so itchy that I could scratch my skin off and have. Times I dream of having a bath, but can't because I will never be able to get out of a tub. The moments when I miss my old life, knowing it will never return.

Sadly, this list could go on for many more pages. To those of us who can add to this list; I find it easier to be content with what I can do rather than pine over what I can't. My future, now that I have one, is something I get to look forward to everyday. Please don't ever take yours for granted.

Not all the choices I have made in my life have been wise ones. But they were all appropriate for me at the time. They taught me valuable lessons and forced me to grow and have faith. Sometimes I look back and wonder how I ever survived. There is a thin line between stubborn and stupid. I tend to cross that line more than I should. A lot of my behavior has made people around me concerned. I understand intellectually where they are coming from, but my heart and spirit are not always on the same page as them.

Not everything I have learned has been easy on me or those around me.

What I have learned, first and foremost, is that I had to be my own health advocate. I have to watch out for myself because I shouldn't rely on anyone else, sometimes it's okay though. I'm lucky I have Kyle, but even still, you should always rely on yourself. Hold onto what little independence you have.

I had to speak up when I needed something. Only YOU truly know what YOU need. Every patient with multiple sclerosis needs to fight their own fight, never take no for an answer for what's best for you. If I want something to change, I alone have the power to make it happen. I just need to voice it.

I've learned to have faith in what I don't understand.

There are harsh truths of who your true friends are, especially when becoming ill. Don't worry, after the sadness there is clarity.

I know that my physical body has a mind of its own. Sometimes it works for me, sometimes it doesn't, but I still have the ability to control how I react to this.

I know not all things are as they seem. I have learned much more than I ever thought possible. This life has given me more than I could have ever imagined.

I've been described with many complimentary words. I don't feel deserving of such commendations. I'm still flattered when I receive them but, I haven't done anything incredibly spectacular to survive.

There are many people in this world who are far more deserving of such compliments.

The advice I have to offer for those suffering from MS or supporting loved ones with MS is this:

Try not to take a single day for granted, you never know when it will be taken away. Love deeper, the time we have with our loved ones will never be enough. Show gratitude, don't just say it.

Never give up.

For every action, there is a reaction, sometimes it's good, sometimes it's not – don't stress over what's out of your control. The outcome of your life is solely up to you. Try not to leave too many casualties while you're learning. As the ill ones, no matter the disease, we need to stand together. There is strength in numbers.

So now, I bid you adieu. Know that no matter what transpires in my life, for better or worse, I have gained freedom. Freedom is a word I didn't know the meaning of until I got sober. The word freedom was more profound when I was no longer held hostage by my disease. The freedom gained from the procedure that unrestricted my life, my time. It is almost impossible to explain, but I'll try. I am free to use my fingers when they work well enough so I can tie my shoes or hold cutlery while I feed myself. I have the freedom to wipe my own bottom. I'm free to stand in the shower. Free to cook for my loved ones. Freedom comes in many aspects; it all depends on how you look at it. If I am sick, or unable to do all that I have listed, I'm still free to smile.

## *ACKNOWLEDGEMENTS*

Now it is time for me to give commendations to all those who've stood beside me.

I applaud my parents; there are no others quite like them. Their never-ending support is something truly inspirational. Their love is the only strength that carries me through some days.

I cannot name all who supported me through my sobriety and MS, there are far too many. Please know I love and appreciate everything you've all done for me, you are all my reminders of the good in the world.

Teena, my sister, when you left there was a hole in my heart. This was difficult for me as a youngster. I thank you for all of the birthday parties and our precious moments. Thank you for your support today, for the friendship that grows a little more each day.

Never to be overlooked is my dearest Ralph. I'm not sure who I would be today without his unwavering support and valuable advice. Ralph was the man who stood in front of me when I needed a tow, behind me when I needed a push, and beside me when I was on even ground. Rest easy sweet Ralph, you are one in a million.

For Alisha, she became my nearest and dearest with all her help on this journey. Alisha, without you none of this would be happening. I was stranded between knowing this needed to be done and the fear of not being able to. With your immense help, love, and endurance, we are here. I thank you.

To my dear Ann, without your dedication to your career and all the people you fought for everyday over 25 years with the Society, I would not be here. You did many amazing things for me in the time that you knew me. I thank you and I miss you. I know that retirement is bittersweet, thanks for saving me before you left us.

In the Crowsnest Pass, I wish to extend thanks to all those who took care of me when my illness had progressed past taking care of myself. For my friends in the city that stood beside me, please know how dear I hold you all in my heart. All my friends on the highway that came to rescue me on more than one occasion THANK YOU.

I wish to extend gratitude to all of my employers since my illness. I would never have made it through without them. The tolerance and understanding of Jayco International and Bison Transport is unsurpassed.

There aren't enough Thanks to the Multiple Sclerosis Societies of Lethbridge, Calgary and Red Deer. I thank Lethbridge for being pivotal in their research, for following Dr. Freedman and his Stem Cell research. I am thankful to Red Deer for being here now, during my recovery. Thanks to Calgary for so much of their time.

Special acknowledgments for the Lethbridge Day Medicine staff who administered my monthly infusions of Cyclophosphamide.

It is absolutely essential I give thanks to the main doctors who dealt with my Autologous Stem Cell Replacement, also known by its proper name Hematopoietic Stem Cell Transplant.

First being Dr. Mark Freedman of the Ottawa General Hospital Multiple Sclerosis Clinic, if not for this man I would not be writing this to you. Secondly, Dr. Harold Atkins who is as important as Dr. Freedman, he is the head Hematologist that performed my transplant. Dr. Atkins was the head of a team of nurses and doctors that took the best care of me during the scariest time in my life. There are three nurses I have fond memories of while in Ottawa. Marjorie Bowman, Dr. Freedman's right hand and Katie Lucas, who is the liaison between the Multiple Sclerosis Clinic, the Hematology team, and me. Katie was the go to lady in all matters once I was in the transplant regime protocol. She was there for absolutely any question I had pretty much whenever I had one.

Linda Hamlin, the nurse who was in my room the entire day of the transplant. She is the last person I remember seeing the day I had my new cells placed back in my body. The rest of the Ottawa General Hospital, I cannot say enough. All the amazing people on the fifth floor with your patience and kindness, you will always close be to my heart. I have admiration for the entire staff of ladies in Day Medicine, where I received hours of Chemotherapy. I am incredibly grateful for the Canadian Blood Bank personnel that were all smiles on days I felt like dying. Many thanks go to all of the terrific staff at the hospital Tim Horton's, and the CHEO Oasis staff for becoming our family away from home. For our beautiful friends Neil and Joan Bushe who became my Ottawa parents, your friendship is a blessing I cherish.

I wish I could name everyone but I know I am unable to remember them all. There is nothing that would hurt my heart more than overlooking someone.

Dr. Baljinder Mann, my General Practitioner in Calgary before moving to the Crowsnest Pass where Dr. Peter McKernan of the Bellvue Medical Clinic took over my day to day care. They are both the most phenomenal practitioners that a person in my shape could have asked for. For all nursing staff, there are no words for the inspiring, painstakingly awesome work you all do each day.

To Dr. Richard Baverstock, my Urologist since 2010. Dr. Baverstock has spent the last many years Botoxing my bladder to ease as much agony as possible. I thank him for doing all that he has to make my life as pleasant as can be.

I'd like to make a special acknowledgment for Dr. Dawn Pearson, my neurologist who works out of the Calgary South Campus Multiple Sclerosis Clinic. Dr. Pearson has taken care of me for the last nine years. We battled MS together. Dr. Pearson fought for years to do all she was able to help me. She fought for me until she had no choice but to turn the reigns over to Ottawa. I commend Dr. Pearson for not putting up barriers that would have made the process more difficult, there are many doctors that do.

I need to give kind regards to the Multiple Sclerosis Clinic at the Foothills Hospital. The first eight years I saw Dr. Pearson was out of this Clinic. My nurse Kathy Billesberger at the Foothills Multiple Sclerosis Clinic cannot be over looked. She is a woman who held my hand and listened when I cried. She was there from the very beginning. In 2005 she explained my disease to me. Kathy explained over and over again how ill I was.

I refused to listen until the day she said outright, "Fiona you are dying. You need to figure this out." From that day forth I did. I finally heard what people had been saying for a long time. Thank you for this Kathy.

To Kyle, last but certainly not least. Your love and patience with me and my disease has been nothing short of astounding. I have learned so much from your silent belief in me. You are a pillar of strength and compassion. If I didn't have you, I know I wouldn't be alive today. Nothing I do will ever repay you for all of the sacrifices you made for me. You are a man of great character and I am grateful for everyday that I have with you. Thank you for being my caregiver, my best friend and my ultimate love story.

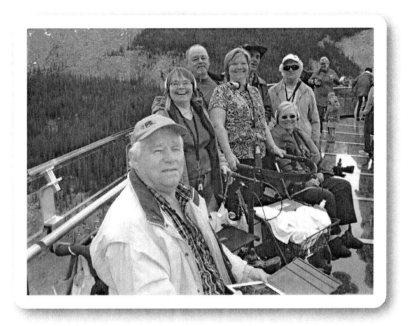

*From left to right My dad, Teena, Kyle, me, mom, Grandpa Jones and Auntie Betty at the Glacier Skywalk in Jasper National Park*

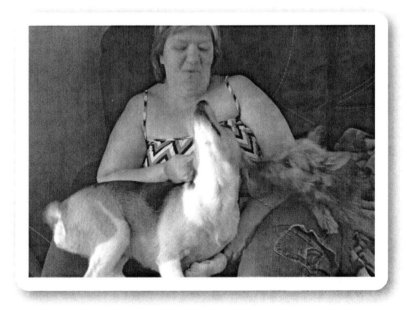

*Me, Itchy and Licr*

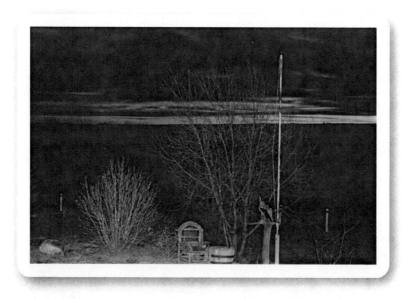

*This is my home, what I am blessed with everyday*

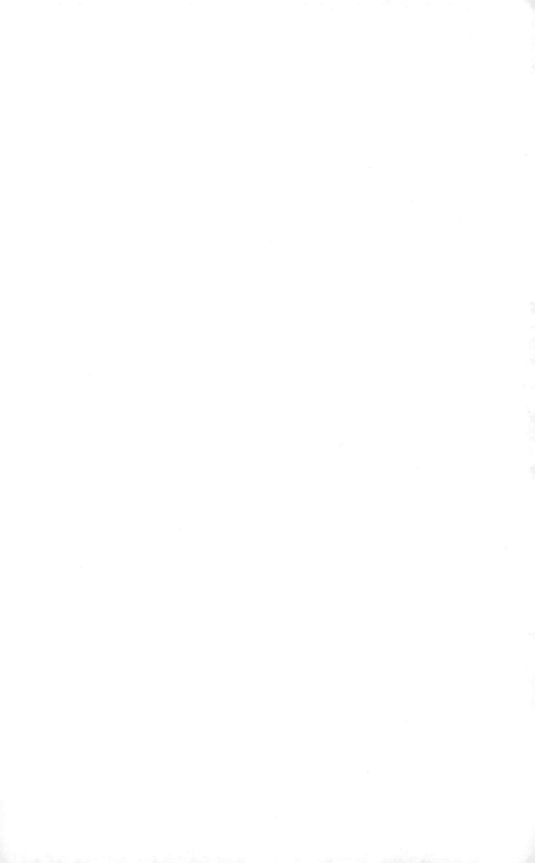

CPSIA information can be obtained at www.ICGtesting.com
Printed in the USA
LVOW07s0516150415

434581LV00005B/80/P